This manual is not affiliated with the U.S. Military. It is intended as an educational tool devised to keep you informed of the latest medical knowledge. It is not intended to serve as a substitute for changing the treatment advice of your doctor. You should never make a medical change without first consulting with your doctor.

Copyright © 2014 Health Opera Press

ISBN 0-9668709-4-8

Published by:

Health Opera Press, PO Box 1471, Madison, AL 35758. Website: http://www.healthopera.biz. Email: donna@healthopera.biz
Printed in the U.S.A.

Training is available. Call 256-655-1626 or email: donna@healthopera.biz.

Table of Contents

ACKNOWLEDGEMENTS

I want to thank several people who in many ways contributed to this total wellness book. Glenn Reese who tactfully reminded me that the total wellness book was not done which actually led to my starting to the write the book. He really did encourage me to move forward.

Also I want to graciously thank my friends Rob Dewberry and Paul Pressley for all of their support. Deciding the book cover was quite a task for me and with the help of Birchwood, Jennifer, and Nate, I was able to put my thoughts together. In addition the painstaking work of my editor and friend, Shelley Walker, who assisted with putting the icing on the cake – a superb thanks to you.

About the Author

Donna Smith is president of Health Opera, LLC, a nationally recognized health expert and registered dietitian with a Master's degree in Public Health from Loma Linda University, Loma Linda, CA. She started her company, Health Opera, so individuals can access credible seminars and resources from one source.

Ms. Smith has consulted for universities, private organizations, churches, corporations, television (Channel 19 News, 3ABN) and radio broadcasts (WOL, WJOU, WLOR, WGCR.US). Her weekly radio program *Sound Advice with Donna Smith* was a hit with topics ranging from good eating to dating.

She also served as a professor and director of the dietetics program at Oakwood University and is currently working for the military as a nutritionist. It was during this time that she realized the drastic need for a step-by-step practical and completely encompassing wellness approach that benefits both military service members and civilians.

ARMY WELL – 8 Steps to Total Wellness is one of several books on health that Ms. Smith has authored. One of her books made the best seller list in its category on Amazon. She was also most delighted when her macaroni *n' cheese* recipe won the taste-testing contest and was published in the very first issue of **Real Health** magazine.

Today she promotes **ARMY WELL** - **8 Steps to Total Wellness** program emphasizing strong bodies, strong minds, and social well-being. In this program you will learn the fitness life skills necessary to increase your fit factor and really move forward with living.

Welcome

This lifestyle manual is designed to assist you with achieving optimal health and wellness. By following the principles of each acronym (ARMY WELL) you can move forward to embrace a purposeful life while experiencing improved appearance, energy, physical and mental stamina.

Old behaviors lead to old results, and the steps to gain new behaviors are detailed in an easy format for busy people to grasp. Carefully review each section to determine your state of readiness for that new behavior. It is best to take small steps and blend these into your current lifestyle.

Everything outlined is reasonable, reliable and achievable. Focus on what you want to achieve. This program includes all 8 steps needed for total wellness. Total wellness is necessary for enhanced physical performance. Start today to begin your fantastic journey toward a healthier life in the fit lane!

Motto:

You're not well unless you're

ARMY WELL

A – Air
R – Rest
M – Meal Planning
Y – Yield
W – Water
E – Exercise
L – Longevity
L – Leisure

Introduction

ARMY WELL – 8 Steps to Total Wellness is designed for active military, reservist, retired military or civilians. Increase your fit factor by incorporating the **ARMY WELL** principles outlined. If you are reading this book you want change. You want to take charge of your life and feel the good results.

This is a straight-forward approach to health and wellness with no bells or whistles. It is important to familiarize yourself with all steps and determine your starting point.

Total wellness is not a race but a lifestyle. Sometimes we give up too soon because it's not comfortable. It takes about 20 days to break a habit. Give yourself room to feel a little uncomfortable before throwing in the towel.

There are eight steps to get you moving into the fit lane. Adapt these steps toward your current lifestyle or situation. Soldiers in a combat zone obviously may not have the option of doing all 8 steps to the degree outlined.

Do what you can and share the information with your family and friends. Civilians will have more flexibility and fewer challenges.

No magic pill, lotion or cream can zap you into good health. Following the latest trendy diet or highly advertised health gimmicks is a true waste of time. It's back to basics with sound advice that works! Poor health costs time, energy and money.

I am often amazed when clients tell me how much better they feel or how they are losing weight, and all they did was follow some of the simple steps that I outlined for them. I recommend you follow the principles outlined in each chapter.

Everyday you must make the decision that your health is important to do something about it. Depending upon your effort, persistence, and current physical condition will determine your ultimate results.

Check with your primary physician before embarking on any new physical program. This program is not designed to take the place of your health professional's program. This is information that you can use based on scientific research, personal practice and many years of working with clients, groups and organizations who want better health.

Why should I read ARMY WELL - 8 Steps to Total Wellness?

1. You can get all the necessary components to increase your fit factor in one reference. You learn not only core

information regarding diet and exercise but all 8 steps to improve your health and chances for longevity.

2. I have over 20 years of experience working as a registered dietitian and professor in college teaching students, cancer survivors, diabetics, and heart patients about how to use diet as therapy.

3. It is a useful quick reference with plain simple facts you need to achieve better health.

4. You will receive guides and useful resources to help you plan healthier meals and have tasty recipes.

5. You will learn the importance of how breathing and rest are essential to a healthy foundation.

6. Solid tips to manage stress successfully are clearly outlined. Stress is a powerful de-energizer if not managed.

7. You will learn principles to begin your purposeful life and embrace physical activity to increase your circulation and strengthen your body.

8. You will learn how balance and recreation both rejuvenate you and help you to be more productive.

Your body is wonderfully crafted to work in a precise and harmonious system of complete balance. *ARMY WELL - 8 Steps to Total Wellness* is based upon well-researched information. To function in an orderly balanced system requires several components. You will learn what you need to do to achieve better health.

YOU are
A CUT
above
THE REST

Step 1: Air

Poor indoor air quality has been linked to headaches, fatigue, trouble concentrating, eye irritants, nasal irritants, as well as throat and lung problems. Specific air contaminants along with damp indoor environments affect people suffering from asthma. In addition, asbestos, radon, high or low humidity, recent remodeling, airborne chemicals, mold, and cleaning supplies may all cause poor indoor air quality that is known to affect your health.

Occupational Safety & Health Administration (OSHA) has standards about ventilation and specifications on some of the air contaminants. Unhealthy air quality in stuffy old buildings is a health concern. Why wait for OSHA to check your office building? The best preventive practice is to open the windows or go outside and breathe.

According to Dr. David Williams proper breathing can aid in lowering your blood pressure, detoxifying, thinking more clearly, relieving stress and lowering your heart rate. Proper respiration could certainly benefit our dutiful service members and eliminate some common health effects.

In the winter, we close our windows in our offices, homes and cars to keep the cold outside. In the summer, we close our windows in our offices, homes and cars to keep the cool inside. A basic ingredient to vitality is fresh air.

Your lungs are constantly throwing off impurities, and they need oxygen. Take five deep breaths of morning air to purify your blood. Stand up with shoulders back and put your hands on your stomach. Take a deep breath inhaling through your nose and exhaling through your mouth. Allow your stomach to go out while doing this and hold it for a few seconds then release slowly.

You will be amazed how this simple exercise can rejuvenate your entire body. Instead of the usual coffee break throughout the day, you can do these deep breathing exercises to relax you and oxygenate your whole body.

Open up the window to allow fresh air into the room or go outside if you can't open the window. You may find this difficult to do on cold winter days but it is necessary all year long. Fresh air is extremely important to your total wellness.

Here's the Deal!

Shallow breathing limits the amount of oxygen your body needs. It's as if you go to your ATM machine and have thousands of dollars to spend but you can only extract $30.00. Obviously, this limits your buying power. This total wellness program is designed to empower you.

Every cell in your body needs rich oxygen. I often sit slumped in my chair at the computer. I intentionally take several breaks at work and at home practice my posture exercises.

If a few simple practices can improve your health and make you feel alive, then I encourage you to invest your time taking deep breaths first thing in the morning and definitely throughout the day.

Your Next Step: Rest

Notes and Action:

_____

_____

_____

_____

_____

_____

_____

_____

_____

_____

_____

_____

_____

_____

ARMY WELL

Deep breathing reduces stress and improves your overall well-being

Step 2: Rest

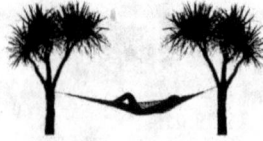

Good quality sleep is necessary to maintain mental and physical performance. You are better equipped to handle decisions, calculate varying operations, possess the stamina to execute tasks and filter your communications. Oftentimes, words hastily spoken and feelings of irritability are the result of insufficient sleep.

An estimated 50 to 70 million Americans suffer from sleep disorders. Sleep disorders are changes in sleeping patterns or habits, and symptoms include excessive daytime sleepiness, irregular breathing, restless sleep, difficulty sleeping, and abnormal sleep behaviors.

If you suffer from this disorder you should seek medical attention to get an accurate diagnosis. Whether you have a diagnosed sleep disorder or routinely get little sleep due to a packed schedule, inadequate rest can affect your overall health, safety and quality of life. Service members particularly must address any issues that impact their rest.

Long-term effects of sleep deprivation have been associated with an increased risk of hypertension, diabetes, obesity, heart attack, and stroke. Let's take a closer look at two of the long-term effects of inadequate sleep mentioned, diabetes and obesity.

Diabetes

Researchers have viewed evidence from cross-sectional studies, and they determined that an increase in diabetes risk may be due to little or poor quality sleep. Insufficient sleep alters insulin resistance, which is associated with an increased risk of developing type 2 diabetes. Insulin resistance is like having an ATM card with the correct code and plenty of money in your account, but the code is not recognized. Frankly, who needs that type of resistance?

With increased prevalence of diabetes alone, it is good to know that something as simple as getting more rest could possibly prevent this chronic illness.

Obesity

Obesity is associated with short sleep duration. Lack of sleep affects hormones that regulate satiety and hunger. An imbalance of these hormones means your gauge to eat and how much to eat is off. You need that gauge so you won't eat the whole pie plus.

This is why total wellness includes simple rest. A well-rested body lays the foundation for great health. Our society is overstimulated. The internet, social media, sports and excessive negative news reports interfere with your getting sound rest. Most people require 7 – 8 hours of quality sleep.

Sleep Cycles

Sleep occurs in cycles and consists of two basic states: Rapid Eye Movement (REM) and Non Rapid Eye Movement (NREM). The REM cycle is light sleep and your eyes move rapidly, and your breathing becomes more irregular and shallow. During NREM your body shifts through stages 1 - 4. Stages 3 and 4 are deeper levels of sleep needed to rejuvenate you and build bones and muscles.

Quality sleep requires several components

1. Comfort – Invest in a supportive mattress.

2. Melatonin – Sleep is regulated by the hormone melatonin. Producing melatonin requires a dark room, so make sure you turn off all lights, including lights from computers and television.

3. Time – Go to bed a few hours before midnight to have several hours of producing the needed melatonin.

4. Satiety – Eat a serving of carbohydrates a few hours before bedtime. A slice of toast, cucumber, apple, small bowl of cereal banana are good sources of carbohydrates.

5. Relax – Avoid stressful activities prior to bed and de-stress by enjoying a warm bath, reading an inspiring book or listening to soft, quiet music. Also, avoid consuming caffeine several hours before bedtime.

6. Routine – Establish a bedtime routine to get you in the mood for winding down.

7. Air - Open a window allowing fresh air into the room where you sleep.

Here's the Deal!

Benjamin Franklin was an US author, politician, writer, physician, and inventor who quoted, "Early to bed and early to rise makes a man healthy, wealthy, and wise." I would definitely take the advice of a man who has accomplished so much.

Obviously, active soldiers do not have the luxury of always determining their bedtime. However, when in a situation to go to bed at a certain time do not neglect this for unnecessary activities. If you work the graveyard shift and sleep during the day, create as dark a room as possible. Remember producing the hormone melatonin, which regulates sleep, requires a dark room.

No computer lights, night lights or glares from the television should be seen. Sleeping in a dark room may seem weird in the beginning but keep doing it until it becomes more comfortable. Simple practices can make a big difference in the quality of your health and life. Manufacturing healthy hormones requires quality sleep.

Your Next Step: Meal Planning

Notes and Action:

_____

_____

_____

_____

_____

_____

_____

_____

_____

_____

_____

_____

_____

_____

_____

_____

_____

ARMY WELL

The body's best medicine is a good sound sleep

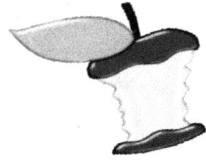

Step 3: Meal Planning

In this section, meal planning tips based on simple pointers and easy guides will help you plan nutritious meals. In addition, some recipes and resources for more healthy menus are provided. It takes just a little time to prepare healthier meals, but it is worth the time.

Planning meals saves money, patience, time at home and time at the grocery store. Proper meal planning and eating right can help you maintain a healthy body weight. According to a study utilizing data on health behaviors among military personnel, the U.S. military is experiencing a trend toward being overweight not explained by a decrease in physical activity.

Maintaining a healthy body weight is essential if you are in the military and still important if you are not. Also, the prevalence of eating disorders is increasing among active duty soldiers. The pressure to maintain the proper weight is stressful unless you practice healthy meal planning. Think fitness for life and eat items that you enjoy but keep it healthy.

Healthy meal planning also include the spices and flavor enhancers you like to use. Try a variety of herbs or your own spice blends to dress up your meal. Remember it takes time for your taste buds to make adjustments.

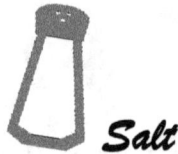

Salt

Salt is added to food as a preservative and a flavor enhancer. Since salt is an acquired taste, you will have to painstakingly reduce using a lot over a period of time. You can make the adjustment and still enjoy your food.

> **Note:** Consult your doctor before using any salt substitute.

Try fresh ingredients such as parsley, basil, thyme or cilantro to add flavor to your food. Any seasoning that is in a powder form is alright to use. For example, you can use onion powder versus onion salt to enhance your food. Add salt after you cook the food to reduce the amount you use.

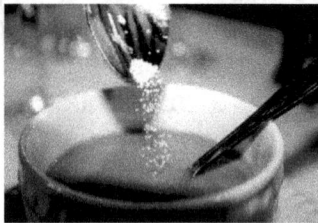

Sugar

Sugar is also a flavor enhancer. Whether you choose one lump or two while preparing food, make sure you note the amount you use. Every teaspoon of sugar is approximately 16 calories and the calories add up easily.

Natural ingredients such as dates, raisins, or fruit can be used as sweeteners. These natural ingredients really add sweetness and usually are fewer calories than table sugar. Diabetics must be careful about the use of natural sweeteners and should consult your dietitian for proper meal planning.

Amount	Food Item	Calories
1 cup	Dates	415
1 cup	Raisins	434
1 cup	Sugar, granulated	774

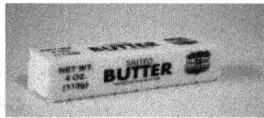

Fat

Using fat such as butter, margarine, salad dressing, gravy, cheese sauce, mayonnaise or cream cheese adds significant calories. It's a taste adjustment to learn to enjoy food without all of the additional high calorie toppings.

Be careful consuming low fat versions of regular rich toppings because the tendency is to eat more. Manufacturers of low fat foods or substitutes add more sugar or salt to enhance their flavor. Try substituting low fat yogurt versus sour cream as a topping for some food items.

Amount	Food Item	Calories
1 tablespoon	Mayonnaise	94
1 tablespoon	Butter	102
1 tablespoon	Margarine	102
1 tablespoon	Sour Cream	23
1 tablespoon	Ranch Salad Dressing	63

Here are the more basic meal planning tips for you and your family. Keep it simple and follow these guidelines:

Eyes – Make meals attractive by using nice dinnerware or garnishes such as tomato wedges, fresh parsley or baby carrots. Use colorful foods which are a natural eye grabber.

Nutrition – Select foods that provide the six nutrients (carbohydrate, protein, fat, vitamin, mineral, water) your body needs to function properly. Choose a wide variety of foods. Eat from all of the basic food groups (dairy, protein, fruit/vegetable, grain).

Adequacy – Choose a diet that provides enough calories and nutrients to meet your physical needs. Sometimes feeling tired, irritable, weak or getting sick frequently can result from not getting enough nutrients.

Plan ahead – Try doing the chopping, cutting, slicing, or pre-preparation in the morning and then assemble the food and cook it in the evening. Also consider one or two days to do bulk cooking. Place the food into smaller containers designed for freezing and make your own homemade TV dinners.

Save $$$ – Be creative with leftovers and not let them go to waste. Cook what's in season and what's on sale. Be careful with coupons, you may spend more if you are buying a lot of items you don't need or ordinarily use.

Planning healthy, tasty menus is fun and worth the effort. You don't have to be a nutrition expert or gourmet chef to plan and enjoy wholesome meals.

Use the My Plate food planning guide to help ensure you get all the nutrients you need. This is just a general guide because in some circumstances you may need more servings than recommended from a particular food group. The main emphasis is to eat from all of the food groups.

For more useful information on meal planning tips and good nutrition, visit these websites: www.MyPlate.gov. or www.healthopera.biz.

My Plate – A Food Planning Guide

Food Group	Some Nutrients Provided
Dairy Group (2 - 3 servings/2 to 3 cups)	Calcium, Protein, Vitamin B12, Vitamins A & D (when fortified) **Food Sources:** Milk, yogurt, cottage cheese, cheese, broccoli, tofu, Bok Choy, almonds, turnip greens, kale
Protein Group (2 servings/5 - 6 ounces)	Protein, Iron, Phosphorus, Vitamin B6, Vitamin B12, Magnesium, Niacin **Food Sources:** Meat, nuts, tofu, beans, eggs
Fruits/Vegetables (5 -13 servings/ 2 ½ cups to 6 ½ cups)	Vitamin A, Vitamin C, Potassium, Magnesium, Folate **Food Sources:** Most orange and yellow fruits/vegetables, kiwi, bananas, citrus fruits, potatoes, dark green leafy vegetables
Grains breads, cereals, pancakes, pasta, muffins, biscuits – 6 to 8 ounces 1 slice bread, 1 cup ready-to-eat cereal, or ½ cup cooked rice pasta or cereal can be considered as 1 ounce equivalent	B1, B2, B3, Iron, Protein, Magnesium **Food Sources:** Corn, whole wheat, rye, oats or oatmeal, brown rice, barley, millet, bulgur, couscous

Food Purchasing

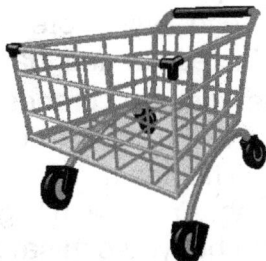

Careful planning and buying helps you to save money and time. It can also reduce waste and help improve the quality of meals prepared.

Successful food buying depends on purchasing good quality foods at the best prices. Purchasing the correct quantities can also reduce food costs. Buying in bulk usually saves money unless food spoils because it has expired.

I always have to be careful especially with my fresh produce. I try to wash it and cut it up and place it in an airtight container as soon as I bring it home. How often have you thrown fresh fruits and vegetables away because they rotted right in your refrigerator? This certainly is not a good way to save dollars.

You may also consider freezing fresh produce if you do not plan to use them soon. The key is to have a plan that works for you.

Note: Buying foods in season see Appendix A – Meal Planning III. Seasonal Food Purchasing

Tips for saving pennies:

- ✪ Don't shop when you are hungry. The tendency to buy more or compulsive buying increases and that adds $$$.
- ✪ Consider store brands. Oftentimes they have the same quality as brand names. The main difference is in the packaging. You won't get the fancy wrapping but you can save $$$.
- ✪ Check your household inventory of food items before you go shopping so you won't buy what you already have.
- ✪ Focus on fresh produce in season and you also get better quality as well as save $$$.
- ✪ Consider items above and below eye level. These products are just as nutritious, but may cost less.
- ✪ Buy perishable foods such as meats, fish, and poultry in quantities that can be safely stored in the refrigerator and freezer.
- ✪ The best quality fruits are U.S. Fancy or U.S. No.1. They contain the highest standard of color and an absence of blemishes. Use this grade when you want the fruits to be visible such as in a fruit salad.
- ✪ Purchase frozen foods that have been kept frozen. Do not buy partially thawed foods. Frost or the appearance of snow on frozen foods indicates partial thawing. This lessens the quality of the food product.

2-Day Sample Meal Plan Based Upon MyPlate Food Guide

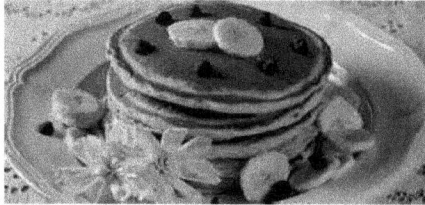

Day 1	Day 2
Breakfast	
Whole Grain Pancakes Fresh Strawberries Milk/Soymilk	Oatmeal Fresh Strawberries Yogurt/Silk Yogurt
Lunch	
Vegetarian Chili* Natural Applesauce Peas Porgy's Hush Puppies*	Macaroni & Cheese* Stewed Tomatoes* Garden Salad Whole Grain Rolls
Dinner	
Baked Fish Brown Rice Green Beans Milk/Soymilk	Spicy Grilled Veggies & Tofu Whipped Potatoes Whole Grain Rolls 100% Grape Juice

* Recipes from *Pumpkin's Veggie Delights* and *Finger Lickin' Way to Fight the Fat* (see Resources Section)

Try these simple recipes

(Healthy Breakfast/Lunch Ideas)

Orange Julius   Yield: 3 servings

1-6 oz. frozen orange juice concentrate
1½ cups soymilk
½ cup crushed pineapple
1 tablespoon evaporated cane juice or raw
  sugar
1 teaspoon imitation vanilla

Combine all ingredients in blender. Blend until smooth, about 30 seconds.

Calories: 88, Fat: 2.3 grams, Carbohydrate: 13.7 grams, Dietary Fiber: 1.7 grams, Protein: 3.7 grams, Sodium: 15 milligrams

Kiwi-Berry Bisque   Yield: 6 servings

1 cup soymilk
5 kiwis, peeled
1-16 ounce bag frozen strawberries
4 bananas
2-15 ounce cans sliced peaches in juice (do
  not drain)
½ cup raw sugar or fructose
1 teaspoon cardamom
Garnish: slivered almonds and shredded
  coconut, optional

Puree milk, kiwi, ½ strawberries, and two bananas. Pour puréed mixture over sliced bananas, peaches, and remaining strawberries, then add sweetener and cardamom seasoning.

Garnish with slivered almonds and coconut shreds (not included in nutritional analysis).

Calories: 266, Fat: 1.4 grams, Carbohydrate: 67.2 grams, Dietary Fiber: 6.4 grams, Protein: 3.6 grams, Sodium: 0 milligram

Smith, Donna A. Finger Lickin' Way to Fight the Fat. Health Opera Press, 2005.

Rainbow Bean Salad   Yield: 8 –10

2 cups northern beans, cooked
2 cups kidney beans, cooked
2 cups black-eyed peas, cooked
1 ½ - 2 cups Nasoya Creamy Italian
   dressing or Thousand Islands
1 small red pepper, diced
   Salt and cayenne pepper to taste

Cook beans according to directions. Drain beans then mix them all along with red pepper and seasonings. Cover with dressing.

Calories: 208, Fat: 7 grams, Cholesterol: 0 milligram, Sodium: 165 milligrams.

Smith, Donna A. Pumpkin's Veggie Delights. Madison: Health Opera Press, 1998.

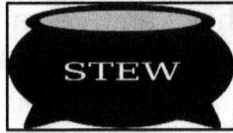

STEW

Lentil Stew   Yield: 6 servings

1-1b dried lentils
½ teaspoon curry powder
1 onion, minced
½ teaspoon cayenne pepper
4-5 bay leaves
4-5 stalks celery, chopped
1 teaspoon cumin
1 tablespoon vegetable oil
½ teaspoon ginger
½ cup fresh parsley chopped
½ teaspoon nutmeg
   Salt to taste

In a large pot prepare lentils according to directions. Sauté onion and celery in a hot oiled skillet. Add onion, celery, bay leaves and seasonings to large pot. Simmer until lentils are well seasoned.

Calories: 207, Fat: 3 grams, Cholesterol: 0 milligram, Sodium: 121 milligrams

Smith, Donna A. Pumpkin's Veggie Delights.
Madison: Health Opera Press, 1998.

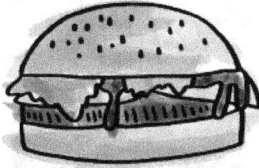

Lentil Burger   Yield: 6-9 patties

¾ cup dried lentils   ½ cup onion, chopped
3 cups water   1 teaspoon salt
1 cup Italian bread crumbs
1 teaspoon sage
¾ cup Egg Beaters
¾ teaspoon thyme
2 teaspoons naturally brewed soy sauce
¼ teaspoon rosemary
   Dash cayenne pepper

Wash and drain lentils. Place lentils and water in saucepan and bring to a boil. Reduce heat and let simmer for 45 minutes or until lentils are tender. Remove from heat, drain, and let cool. Add bread crumbs, eggs, onions, and seasonings to lentils. Mix well. Shape into patties and fry in oil on hot skillet. Cook both sides until done in the middle.

Calories: 139, Fat: 3 grams, Cholesterol: 0 milligram, Sodium: 451 milligrams.

Smith, Donna A. Pumpkin's Veggie Delights. Madison: Health Opera Press, 1998.

Eating on the run!!!

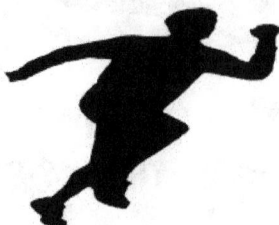

The best plan is to have one. If you don't plan and prepare your meals then what you see is what you get. Dining at work or fast food places oftentimes doesn't leave you with the best food options. When you are in situations with limited healthy selections, I suggest following these simple tips:

1) Most eating places have vegetables and salads which make good choices

2) Choose smaller portions

3) Request baked items vs. fried

4) Request gravies and dressings be placed on the side (use only half)

5) Choose oil salad dressings over creamy salad dressings or better yet freshly squeezed lemon juice

6) Limit desserts

7) Choose fresh fruit in season for a dessert

8) Yogurts are high in sugar unless you discard some of the fruit sauce

9) Drink lemon water or herbal tea vs. beverages

10) Skip the bread if you know your main entrée is high in calories and fat

11) Skip ordering an appetizer if the main entrée is high in calories and fat

12) Only eat a half serving and request the remaining for take-out

13) Choose a hot beverage such as spicy herbal tea instead of an appetizer

14) Request the server not bring any bread or complimentary appetizers

Here's the Deal!

There's a lot of information in this section. Get familiar with the meal planning guides and use them to make sure you are eating from all food groups.

If you always eat out, then definitely familiarize yourself with the previous eating on the run tips. When you don't have the best choices, make the best of the choices you do have. The same rules apply if you are deployed, away for training or in a situation where you can't prepare your own meals.

You have to be intentional about good health. It is not a by-product of negligence. Be flexible, be prepared for those off days, maximize your food value by following the tips in food purchasing, and try the recipes. There are more guides and information in the appendices.

Your Next Step: Yield

Notes and Action:

_____

_____

_____

_____

_____

_____

_____

_____

_____

_____

_____

_____

_____

_____

_____

_____

ARMY WELL

Healthy meals build strong minds and bodies

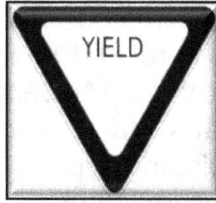

Step 4: Yield

You know you should not yield to certain yummy foods but they are so seducing. You truly have tried many times, only to be back in the same rut. When you see a "yield" sign you slow down and take caution. In this section, I will cover sound advice regarding misuse and excessive indulgences of substances that limit and don't empower you.

I won't cover all of the "nitty gritty", but I will give you enough information to help you make reasonable adjustments to have more control. Use the knowledge to make daily choices toward your journey and pursuit toward total wellness.

You will have difficult decisions to make in this section. The choices you make will determine your outcomes. Those outcomes can reduce your risk of getting diabetes, cardiovascular disease, hypertension, obesity and cancer.

Sugar

Is sugar bad for you? Sugary drinks are a major contributor to obesity. The nation spends an estimated $190 billion yearly treating obesity-related health issues. Also people who drink sugary beverages regularly such as 1 to 2 cans daily have a 26% greater risk of developing type 2 diabetes than people who rarely drink them.

In addition to diabetes, regularly drinking high sugary beverages can increase your chances of heart attacks. Other studies have linked sugar, particularly fructose, with high blood pressure and kidney disease. Whether you consume sugar from beverages or food, it is clear that regularly enjoying delicious sugar has its consequences.

To help you stay on track, follow the sugar guidelines. The recommendations are no more than 9 teaspoons or 36 grams for men and 6 teaspoons or 24 grams for women. A bowl of the average sweetened cereal contains (11 grams sugar) and a honey bun (15 grams) which is a total of 26 grams of sugar and that's just breakfast! Women would have exceeded the goal by 2 grams in just one meal.

Sugar is in snacks, crackers, condiments, cereals, soups, breads, and of course the amount you add from the sugar bowl or packets. No wonder we are having a difficult time keeping within the recommendations.

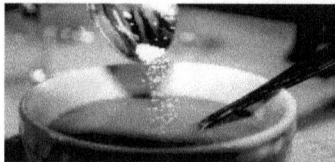

Food manufacturers are adding more sweeteners to our food and you have to be a sugar detective to find them all. Carefully read your labels to locate the sugar content. Ingredients are listed in a descending order meaning those listed first are the majority in that food product.

Here are some common sweeteners:

- ✪ Brown sugar – molasses is added to white sugar
- ✪ Corn syrup – a syrup, mostly glucose, some maltose derived from corn
- ✪ Dextrose – another name for glucose
- ✪ Fructose – the sugar in fruit
- ✪ High fructose corn syrup – mostly fructose and corn syrup
- ✪ Honey – glucose and fructose produced by enzymatic digestion, by bees, of the sucrose in nectar
- ✪ Maple syrup – a concentrated solution of sucrose deived from maple trees, mostly sucrose
- ✪ Molasses – a syrup made from sugar cane, a thick, brown syrup
- ✪ Raw sugar – the first crop of crystals from sugar processing, not sold jn United States, raw sugar in the U.S. is more refined
- ✪ Sucrose – fructose and glucose linked togther, white table sugar
- ✪ Turbinado – raw sugar with some of the debris removed is legal to sell in the United States

The trend today is to satisfy that devilish sweet tooth by using other sweeteners. There is a lot of controversy with some of the sugar substitutes. Sugar substitutes are used in place of sucrose (sugar). They can be placed in two categories (natural and artificial).

Natural sugar substitutes include but are not limited to agave nectar, coconut palm sugar, honey, monk fruit, sorbitol, stevia and xylitol. These sugars are not processed with lots of synthetic materials. They come from plants or sugar alcohols. Don't be concerned, sugar alcohols contain no alcohol (ethanol) and are less sweet than regular sugar.

Alternative sugar substitutes are chemically processed. They are also classified as non-caloric sweeteners because they have no or very little calories. Diabetics and people who are trying to reduce calories are attracted to these sweeteners due to their having little or no calories.

However, there is controversy about their usage. Some alternative sweeteners include aspartame, acesulfame potassium, neotame, saccharin, and sucralose. Health concerns regarding the alternative sugar substitutes include causing cancer in animals, headaches, dizziness, and neurological symptoms.

Center for Science in the Public Interest (CSPI) an advocacy group for nutrition, health, food safety, alcohol policy and sound science, want the Food and Drug Administration (FDA) to conduct more studies to ascertain more certainty regarding their safety.

Review the sugar substitute chart to become more familiar with some of the popular sweeteners on the market today.

Natural Sugar Substitutes

Product	Comments
Agave nectar	Comes from a plant that grows in southwestern U.S. and some parts of South America. They can also make tequila from this same plant. **Health Concerns:** Agave is high in fructose having a low-glycemic index versus glucose which affects your blood sugar. This is why many diabetics are using it. There's not a lot of research to support it being better than other sugars. Some experts say the high amount of fructose in Agave can affect how your body releases a hormone called leptin.

	Leptin is needed to control your appetite. Moreover, too much fructose can lead to high levels of triglycerides or fats. The American Diabetes Association recommends limiting all sources of sugars including Agave.
Coconut palm sugar	Coconut sugar is the dehydrated sap from the coconut palm. It contains the same calories as regular sugar and a few trace minerals and vitamins. You get small amounts of phytonutrients. This low glycemic sugar is better than regular sugar because it doesn't spike your blood sugar levels as high which can lead to serious consequences for diabetics. **Health Concerns:** Coconut palm sugar is not a miracle food and it contains the same amount of calories as sugar. You should limit all sugars because calories add up, and too many calories are a health concern.
Honey	Honey contains trace amounts of vitamins and minerals. It is high in fructose and may not raise your blood sugar as fast as other sweet products.

	Health Concerns: Honey is not sugar free. It is 21 calories per teaspoon and regular sugar is 16 calories per teaspoon. Infants younger than 1 year old should not be fed honey because it could contain a bacteria known as *Clostridium* that causes infant botulism. Infant botulism causes muscle weakness and severe breathing problems.
Monk fruit (Luo Han Guo, Lo Han Kuo)	This sweetener is about 200 times sweeter than sugar. Like artificial sweeteners and stevia leaf extracts, monk fruit extract can be used in a wide range of foods and beverages. It is made from a fruit in China. There has not been good testing done in animals. Center for Science in the Public Interest (CSPI) recommends: Caution using this product
Sorbitol	Less calories than regular sugar and Sorbitol doesn't cause tooth decay. You usually find this sugar substitute in gums, candies or other sugar-free products marketed to diabetics.

	Health Concerns: Sorbitol contains fewer calories than table sugar. Eating a lot can increase your blood sugar, and cause bloating and diarrhea. The American Diabetes Association recommends consuming sugar alcohols in moderation. CSPI recommends: Use caution with this product
Stevia (Truvia)	An extract from the stevia plant and is zero calories. The FDA approved only a refined version of the whole plant. It has a slight aftertaste similar to licorice. **Health Concerns:** A group of UCLA toxicologists wrote a letter to the FDA stating some of their lab tests showed the sweetener to cause mutations and DNA damage and urged further testing. More testing is needed. CSPI currently recommends it's safe to use.
Xylitol	Less calories than regular sugar and it doesn't contribute to tooth decay. You usually find this sugar substitute in gums, candies or other sugar-free products marketed to diabetics.

	Health Concerns: Although it contains fewer calories than table sugar it is not calorie-free. Eating a lot can increase your blood sugar and cause bloating and diarrhea. American Diabetes Association recommends consuming sugar alcohols in moderation. CSPI recommends: Caution using this product

Artificial Sugar Substitutes

Product	Comments
Aspartame (Equal, NutraSweet)	Aspartame (Equal) is a chemical combination of two amino acids (phenylalanine and aspartic acid) and methanol. Equal is 200 times sweeter than regular sugar. **Health Concerns:** Some researchers found evidence that aspartame increases the risk of cancer in men and causes cancer in rodents. In addition some users reported having experienced headaches and dizziness. People with phenylketonuria should not use this product

	since it contains the amino acid they cannot break down, which is phenylalanine. CSPI recommends: Avoid this product
Acesulfame Potassium (Sweet One, Sunett)	This sugar substitutes is 200 times sweeter than sugar. It has been used for decades and has little after-taste. **Health Concerns:** FDA reviewed several studies and determined that this sweetener posed no risk to human health. The manufacturer conducted a few long-term animal studies that showed it might be linked to cancer. CSPI urged the FDA to require better testing. CSPI recommends: Avoid or use in moderation
Neotame	Neotame has zero calories and is 7,000 to 13,000 times sweeter than sugar. It has been approved but is rarely used. Sugar or other artificial sweeteners may be mixed with it to compensate for the taste.

	Health concerns: None noted at this time. CSPI recommends: Safe to use
Saccharin (Sweet n' Low)	This artificial sweetener has 0 calories and is 300 times sweeter than sugar. It is generally mixed with aspartame and other newer artificial sweeteners to counteract the bitter aftertaste. **Health concerns:** The U.S. National Toxicology Program's Report on Carcinogens removed saccharin from their list due to a lack of evidence that it caused cancer in humans. It was previously linked with bladder cancer in rats. CSPI recommends: Avoid this product
Sucralose (Splenda)	Sucralose has 0 calories per teaspoon. The taste is well received and it is 600 times sweeter than sugar. Its popularity has tremendously increased in past years. This sweetener can be used in baking.

	Health concerns: Previously, several studies found that it is not a cancer-causing agent. However, it was announced more recently that it caused leukemia in mice. Obviously, more testing is needed. CSPI recommends: Caution for this product

Ways to reduce sugar intake:

- ✪ Read food labels to check the amount of sugar contained
- ✪ Try half the amount of sugar recommended on recipes (this won't alter the taste drastically)
- ✪ Try eating more fruit with its natural sugar to satisfy your "sweet tooth"
- ✪ Instead of regular sodas try half club soda and half 100% fruit juice
- ✪ Use all fruit spreads in baking instead of jams and jellies to add sweetness
- ✪ Substitute applesauce or mashed bananas for half the amount of sugar in recipes
- ✪ Choose breakfast cereals with < 7 grams of sugar unless it contains fruit
- ✪ Decide to have a dessert on the weekends vs. at every meal

Fat

The American Heart Association recommends limiting total fat intake to less than 25 – 35 percent of your total daily calories. Too much fat can increase your risk of heart disease. If you eat a typical diet of 2,000 calories, no more than 700 calories should come from fat.

Too much fat can lead to atherosclerosis. Atherosclerosis happens when fat buildup clogs an artery and blocks blood supply to your organs and tissues. Sometimes your arterial walls can become stiff and less flexible due to damage, and this is called arteriosclerosis.

When you visit your physician and lab work is required, make sure you know the results. It is your health and you need to be in charge working along with your healthcare provider to maintain good health.

Know your numbers:

- ✪ LDL- low density lipoprotein: 70 -130 mg/dL (lower numbers are better)
- ✪ HDL- high density lipoprotein: more than 50 mg/dL (higher numbers are better)
- ✪ Total cholesterol: less than 200 mg/dL (lower numbers are better)
- ✪ Triglycerides: 10 -150 mg/dL (lower numbers are better)

  Note: Lipoproteins transports fat in your body

Your blood lipid or fat levels can fluctuate depending on your diet, exercise, and heredity. A good lab report today may be less than favorable several months from now. Reading food labels to make sure you are eating in the safety zone is an excellent practice. You must be patient and persistent to achieve total wellness.

Fats are necessary for growth, insulation, and energy. You also get a sense of fullness after eating them. There are different types of fats: polyunsaturated, monounsaturated, saturated, trans fat, and cholesterol.

Polyunsaturated fats are usually liquid at room temperature and are associated with reduced risk of heart disease. Examples of polyunsaturated fats are peanuts, seeds, corn, soybeans, and vegetable oils.

Monounsaturated fats are found in a variety of vegetable oils and foods such as olives, avocados, nuts, corn, and rice bran. Studies show that eating a diet rich in these fats could lower your cholesterol and reduce your risk of heart disease.

Saturated fats are solid at room temperature and are linked with higher risks of coronary artery disease. Examples of saturated fats include stick margarine, butter, lard, meats, most cheeses, and bacon.

Trans fats are linked with increased risk of heart disease and are formed during a chemical process called hydrogenation. Some hydrogenated or partially hydrogenated foods include margarine, vegetable shortening, non-dairy creamers, biscuits, sweet rolls, pie crust, pancake mixes, donuts, and snack foods such as chips.

Cholesterol is only found in animal and animal products. Your body makes it too. Foods such as organ meats, shrimp, clams, lobsters, oysters, and eggs contain high amounts of cholesterol.

Example: 2,000 calories (saturated fat intake should be <15 grams), (trans-fatty acids < 2 grams), (polyunsaturated fat 56 – 77 grams) and (total fat <77 grams)

Here are some common foods and their saturated fat content:

Food Item	Fat Grams	Food Item	Fat Grams
1 slice American cheese	5.0	1 donut	5.99
1 cup 2% milk	3.0	3 ounce roasted chicken	3.17
Big Mac	8.3	1 serving pizza	8.5

Trans fat content of some common foods:

Food Item	Fat Grams	Food Item	Fat Grams
Burger King Fries – large	7.0	KFC Pot Pie	8.0
9 Ore-Ida Tater Tots	2.0	1 KFC Biscuit	4.0
Burger King Chicken Sandwich	2.0	Parkay stick margarine – 1 tablespoon	3.0
3 Nabisco Oreos	3.0	1 Dunkin' Donut, cake type	6.0
7 Nabisco Triscuits	2.0	5 Nabisco Ritz Crackers	1.0

Ways to reduce fat intake:

- ✪ Eat more baked, broiled, and boiled foods
- ✪ Trim off excess fat from meats, limit sauces, and gravies
- ✪ Try reduced fat salad dressings and mayonnaise
- ✪ Be careful of snack foods such as chips and baked goods – look to see if they have trans fats or trans-fatty acids
- ✪ Limit trans-fatty acids to less than 1 percent of your total calories
- ✪ Limit saturated fat to less than 7 percent of your total calories
- ✪ Consume more monounsaturated and polyunsaturated fats such as nuts, seeds, corn, vegetable oils and fish

Salt

The sodium portion of salt can (sodium and chloride) negatively affect your blood pressure. Normal blood pressure is 120/80. The top number is the systolic pressure and the lower number is the diastolic pressure. Constant high blood pressure can lead to hardening of the arteries or arteriosclerosis.

The Dietary Guidelines for Americans recommend limiting your daily sodium intake to less than 2,300 milligrams. Most Americans consume 3,400 milligrams. Sodium is in almost any food that comes in a package or can. Read the food labels and note the food additives that contain sodium.

The most common additives that utilize sodium are as follows:

Monosodium Glutamate (MSG)	*Sodium Benzoate*
MSG is a flavor enhancer and gives food a savory taste. Some people have bad reactions to this seasoning. Other ingredients that may contain MSG include hydrolyzed soy protein and autolyzed yeast.	An additive used as a preservative. Sodium benzoate is used in a variety of processed food products and drinks. In some children it may cause hyperactivity.

Sodium Bisulfite	Sodium Caseinate
It is used to prevent discoloration in certain foods such as dried fruit and frozen potatoes. Be very cautious because some people have really severe reactions to the sulfite.	It is used as a whitening and also thickening agent in several milk products such as ice cream, sherbet and coffee creamers.
Sodium Nitrite	Sodium Propionate
It is used for curing meats such as canned meats and sausages. Sodium nitrite is also associated with cancer.	It is used as a preservative in food preventing the growth of mold and some bacteria prolonging the shelf life of food.

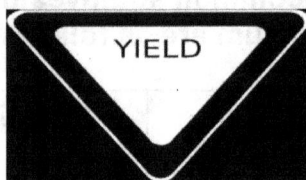

YIELD

Food Item	Sodium Content	Calories
Daily sodium recommendation is 2,300 milligrams		
Hardees's Charbroiled Chicken Club Sandwich	1640 milligrams	610
Panera Bread's Full Bacon Turkey Bravo	2,800 milligrams	800

Taco Bell's Volcano Nachos	1,670 milligrams	970
Wendy's Baja Salad	1,975 milligrams	720
Papa John's Buffalo Chicken Pizza (1 slice)	1,050 milligrams	370
Chipotle's Burrito	2,650 milligrams	1,185
Burger King BK Double Stacker	830 milligrams	520

Ways to reduce salt intake:

- ✪ Limit table salt during food preparation and on cooked food

- ✪ Use a salt substitute (check with your physician some salt substitutes contain potassium)

- ✪ Choose convenience foods sparingly because most are very high in sodium; choose low-sodium or reduced-salt food products

- ✪ Be careful of condiments such as ketchup, pickle relish, olives, mustard, salad dressings, mayonnaise, and barbeque sauces, etc.

- ✪ Use the powder forms of seasonings such as onion powder versus onion salt, garlic powder versus garlic salt or try herbs to season foods

Alcohol and Other Substances

When you drink alcohol, it enters a different pathway than normal digestion and enters the body readily and reaches the brain within a minute. Brain cells are sensitive to alcohol causing them to shrink. The results can lead to irreversible effects on vision, memory, learning, and other important bodily functions.

Service members must perform highly technical tasks requiring mental alertness and good memory. In order to perform well you also need nutrients. Drinking alcohol promotes excretion of important nutrients. Refer to the chart below to see the function of nutrients impaired due to alcohol:

Nutrient	Function
Calcium	Strong bones and teeth, normal muscle contraction
Potassium	Muscle contraction, nerve impulses or performance
Magnesium	Muscle contraction, nerve impulses or performance
Phosphorus	Energy transfer and in cell's genetic material
Zinc	Growth, part of the hormone insulin, wound healing
Thiamin	Used in energy metabolism, supports appetite and nervous system
Folate	Needed to make cells
B-12	Needed to make cells, healthy nervous system

Smoking

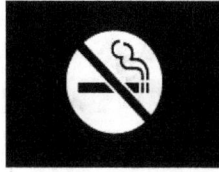

In addition to yielding to alcohol, also include smoking. If you smoke you are walking on thin ice. According to a study in *New England Journal of Medicine*, people who smoke lose at least 10 years of their life expectancy. Those who quit before they are 40 years old reduce the risk of death by 90%, according to the same study.

Smoking is associated with cancer, emphysema and heart disease. When you smoke the compounds in cigarettes produce free radicals which can upset your biological membrane which is a layer that acts as a built-in body guard.

> **Note:** To reinforce these guards you must eat foods high in antioxidants (see Step 7: Longevity for antioxidant food sources).

Smoking decreases powerful antioxidants (vitamin C, vitamin E, carotene and selenium) needed to create your cellular defense. Rarely do you read reports addressing smoking and nutrition.

CAUTION!!

Drugs & Caffeine

Using illegal drugs and the extreme emotional, physical and economic disasters that result can lead to a true life tsunami. Careers, families and lives have been lost due to its use.

Do not underestimate the powerful effect of using caffeine. Caffeine is a drug used to stimulant the central nervous system to make you feel more awake. Some people can't function in the morning without their fix.

Before proclaiming the wonderful alertness you feel after you receive your fix, do note the dark side of caffeine usage.

Carefully review and consider the following negative side effects of caffeine use:

- ✪ Jittery and shaky feelings
- ✪ Makes it hard to fall asleep
- ✪ Makes your heart beat faster
- ✪ Raises your blood pressure
- ✪ Causes headaches, nervousness or dizziness
- ✪ Causes dehydration and can also be addictive

Note: Daily caffeine intake which appears to be safe for most healthy adults should not exceed 400 milligrams. Some experts suggest 200 – 300 milligrams is preferred.

Caffeine content of common foods and drugs are listed below:

Food or Drug	Amount	Caffeine Content in milligrams (mg)
Starbucks Coffee	Venti, 20 fl. oz.	415 mg
Pepsi Max	12 oz.	69 mg
Mountain Dew	12 oz.	55 mg
Pepsi	12 oz.	38 mg
Mr. Pibb	12 oz.	40 mg
Dr. Pepper	12 oz.	41 mg
Coca-Cola	12 oz.	35 mg
5-hour Energy Drink	1.9 fl. oz.	208 mg
Monster Energy Drink	16 fl. oz.	160 mg
Red Bull	8.4 fl. oz.	80 mg
Hershey's Special Dark Chocolate Bar	1.5 oz.	20 mg
Hershey's Milk Chocolate Bar	1.6 oz.	9 mg
No Doz or Vivarin	1 caplet	200 mg
Excedrin Migraine	2 tablets	130 mg

We live in a caffeine craved society and re-gularly rely on its drug-effects to take us beyond our natural abilities. Be aware of your caffeine consumption; it all adds up and can negatively affect your health.

Super-size

Yielding to the bigger the better is a, lose-lose, situation when it comes to some food choices. Super-sized junk food items or sodas provide excessive calories, lots of sugar and fat which can lead to diabetes, obesity, heart disease and other chronic illnesses. You may pay less initially but you pay more in terms of poor health. **Poor health is expensive and can be deadly**.

Portion control is the key to a successful sustained weight control. **An idea of a portion is the size of your fist, computer mouse or a deck of cards.**

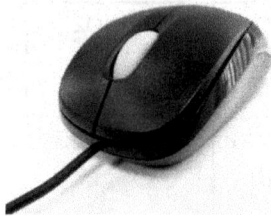

Here's the Deal!

You have committed your life to service and protecting our country. This requires increasing your fit factor and not yielding to things that rob your vitality and life forces.

There's no magic, and it takes patience and persistence to achieve total wellness and increase your fit factor. Trust me it's worth every step to know you are not a slave to cigarettes, alcohol, drugs, and junk food.

No one climbs an entire ladder in one step. One rung at a time and you are on top and that is where I want you to be. You have tried the other gimmiks and they only work temporarily. I am not interested in your investing time and effort for mere temporary results.

Drugs don't fix problems. Substances only numb your reality they do not change it for the better but for worse. Seek professional help to guide you to a safer place.

Your Next Step: Water

Notes and Action:

_____

_____

_____

_____

_____

_____

_____

_____

_____

_____

_____

_____

_____

_____

_____

_____

ARMY WELL

If there is no struggle,
there is no progress.

Frederick Douglas

Practice Exercise I

The answers are in Appendix B.

1. Record what you have eaten for an entire day. Refer to the meal planning guide to compare your results.

2. What are the two basic stages of sleep?

3. Melatonin a healthy hormone is mainly produced during the daylight. (True or False)

4. Carbohydrates, vitamins, minerals, _____, _____, and _____, are the 6 nutrients your body needs:
   a. Water, fat and protein
   b. Phytochemicals, water and protein
   c. Fiber, water and protein
   d. Fiber, water and fat

5. Sugar recommendations are 9 teaspoons or 36 grams for men and 6 teaspoons or 24 grams for women. (True or False)

6. Which of the following are significant food sources of Trans fat:
   a. Potato chips, stick margarine, partially hydrogenated fats
   b. Soybean oil, nuts, corn
   c. Baked goods, stick margarine, potatoes
   d. Hydrogenated fats, corn, nuts, potato chips

7. Smoking cigarettes can lessen your absorption of vitamin C, vitamin E, carotene and selenium which are powerful antioxidants. (True or False)

8. Eating too much sugar can lead to diabetes, osteoporosis, heart disease, cancer and obesity. (True or False)

9. Most experts agree that your daily caffeine intake should not exceed:

   a. 1000 milligrams
   b. 800 milligrams
   c. 400 milligrams
   d. None of the above

10. Recommended sodium intake is less than 2300 milligrams. (True or False)

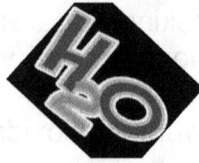

Step 5: Water

It's nonnegotiable. You need it. Every system in your body depends on water. Almost 60% of your body weight consists of water. It flushes toxins out of vital organs, carries nutrients to cells, lubricates joints, regulates body temperature, and helps improve the elasticity of your skin.

Drinking sufficient water helps you to eliminate properly if you also consume enough fiber. Forcing elimination due to hard dry stools is not good. Plus constipation makes you feel drained and sluggish.

Gradually increase your fiber intake along with increasing your water intake. Water and fiber go together like peanut butter and jelly.

> **Note:** Sources of fiber include legumes, fruits, vegetables, whole grains, nuts and seeds

Power to Perform

I was reading about sports and nutrition and one of the best ways to improve your performance is to drink plenty of water. Check your urine output and if it smells of strong ammonia or is a deep yellow color you are probably not getting enough fluids.

After a good night's sleep start your day with a glass of water and continue drinking throughout the day to make sure you are well hydrated. It probably won't seem so overwhelming drinking throughout the day versus drinking a big gulp all at once.

I know it's a bother to have to visit the bathroom more. However, feel blessed if you are going to the bathroom frequently because your kidneys are functioning properly.

Adults need 1.0 to 1.5 milliliters fluid per kilocalorie. If you consume 1800 calories you need 2700 ml of fluid or approximately 11 cups.*

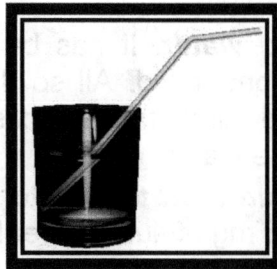

*(240 ml = 1 cup; 2700 ml fluid ÷ 240 ml = 11.25 cups)

Insufficient water drinking can lead to dehydration which is serious and definitely impacts your performance. Keeping well hydrated improves your endurance during physical fitness training.

Please review the following symptoms of both mild to moderate dehydration:

- ✪ Dry, sticky mouth and dry skin
- ✪ Sleepiness or tiredness
- ✪ Thirst
- ✪ Decreased urine output
- ✪ Headache
- ✪ Constipation
- ✪ Dizziness or lightheadedness

The Environmental Protection Agency monitors public water supply and the Food and Drug Administration establishes minimum standards for bottled water. A glossary of water terms is listed below:

- ✪ *Distilled water*. It has been vaporized and recondensed. All solids have been removed and this process produces very pure water.
- ✪ *Fluoridated water*. Water that has at least 0.8 mg of fluoride per liter.
- ✪ *Mineral water*. It contains at least 500 ppm of minerals and is high in sodium.
- ✪ *Natural water*. Water that comes from a spring or well that is regulated to be safe. It also can be filtrated or ozonized.
- ✪ *Public water*. Water from a municipal that has been treated and disinfected.
- ✪ *Purified water*. Water that has been filtered or processed through means such as distillation, reverse osmosis, carbon filtration, and ultra-filtration and other means.

Here's the Deal!

It's one of the basic nutrients your body must have to survive. Water has multiple fundamental functions and getting the correct amounts daily can improve your appearance, mental function and physical performance.

Plain water with no artificial additives is the best. If you don't like the taste of water, try some of the more upscale bottled waters. The different filtering processes applied to them leaves a cleaner taste unlike tap water with the overwhelming taste of chlorine or rust.

Also dilute fruit juice with plain water which is recommended over the alternative sugar substitutes and coloring that are added to flavor water. You can gradually increase the amount of water until you are truly getting much more water than fruit juice.

The more active you are the more water you will need. Also, weather conditions and how much you perspire will ultimately determine the exact amount of water you require.

Your Next Step: Exercise

Notes and Action:

_____

_____

_____

_____

_____

_____

_____

_____

_____

_____

_____

_____

_____

ARMY WELL

Water is the spring of life;
drinking 8 - 11 cups daily
is adequate for most
people.

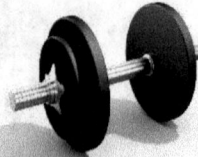

Step 6: Exercise

Sedentary Military/Civilians

There will be times when you are not training or working in the field and your physical demands lessen. Still put exercise on your daily to do list. Be determined and start now even if it is 15 minutes strolling. Do something that works for you. Vary your routine so you won't get bored and plan different activities to work different parts of your body.

Physical activity produces fitness. Being fit enables you to meet the stressful demands of life and reduces risks for certain diseases such as osteoporosis, diabetes, certain types of cancers, high blood pressure and a poor circulatory system.

Gradually increase your physical activity to reduce the chances of bodily injury. Stretch all major body groups (arms, legs, back, shoulders) 5 – 10 minutes, and then walk or run in place to get your muscles warmed up. Include strength training and activities that allow you to be more flexible. If your daily work mainly has you at your desk or you recently suffered an injury, perform office exercises.

Office Exercises

You can still tone and burn calories while at your desk or in your office area. If you are using your muscles you are burning calories and using glucose which is good for diabetics who must keep their blood glucose levels from getting too high. Increasing your heart rate is also a good mind booster and breaks the routine of sitting for long periods which is not good for your circulation.

Always check with your physician before doing any activity especially if you have had an injury or have been inactive.

Take mini-activity breaks and perform some of the following office exercises outlined:

✪ Sit with your back aligned with the back of the chair and extend your legs per-pendicular to the floor. Hold this position and count to 10 and release. Repeat this for 5 times or more. You don't want to strain your back so make sure you are sitting to the back of the chair for support.

✪ Stand up and tip toe and hold that position, then release. Repeat this 5 times or more.

✪ Raise your arms shoulder length and make quick small circular movements forward for several times and then repeat and go backwards for several times.

✪ Sitting with your back aligned to the chair, raise one knee up as high as you can go and then drop. Do this 5 times or more and repeat with the other knee.

✪ Stand up and sit down and repeat this for 5 times or more.

✪ Do several jumping jacks.

✪ Run in place for 60 seconds.

✪ Shadow box for a minute or two.

✪ Do walk-lunges

✪ Twist side to side rapidly for 7 – 10 times

Active Military/Civilians

Start gradually to avoid injury and lactic acid accumulation in the muscles. Lactic acid is produced during anaerobic metabolism. It increases during intense exercise making muscles sore and you produce less when your muscles are more conditioned. Lactic acid goes to the liver to make glucose to fuel you.

Heavy Exercise ⇒	Lactic acid buildup ⇒	Goes to liver ⇒	Liver makes glucose ⇒	Fuels Muscles

Note: Your muscle cells cannot handle too much lactic acid and it goes to the liver to get converted to glucose to fuel your activity. Remember the more conditioned your muscles the less lactic acid produced.

Performance pointers during strenuous exercise:

✪ Eat a high carbohydrate diet approximately 8 grams per kilogram (kg) of body weight or 70% of your caloric intake.

  Note: Carbohydrates are broken down to glucose. Glucose is needed to fuel your muscles and give you energy during exercise.

✪ Protein is required for muscle development. During heavy physical activity your body breaks down protein more. Some experts say you need 1 - 2 grams protein per kilogram (kg) of body weight.

Example Protein Needs

200 lb man = 90.9 (kg)

1 kg = 2.2 lb (200 ÷ 2.2 = 90.9 kg)

90.9 kg x 2 grams protein = 182 grams protein

Note: Protein sources include nuts, seeds, beans, lentils, whole grains, vegetables, dairy, meats, textured vegetable protein (meat substitutes), eggs, tofu, quinoa

---

✪ Eat a wide variety of food (see menu planning and nutrition section for more details). If you eat a wide variety to maintain a healthy weight you are probably getting sufficient protein. Refer to "Example Protein Needs" on page 81 to calculate your protein needs.

✪ Avoid dehydration. Even 2 – 3% body weight loss due to inadequate intake of water will decrease your performance. This represents 6 – 8 cups of body water lost.

✪ Strenuous exercise (3 or more hours) requires replenishing water and sodium losses. Weigh yourself before and after you exercise. If you sweat excessively losing 5 to 10 pounds, then you must replenish your losses.

✪ Drink a sports beverage containing electrolytes or one-third teaspoon salt plus 1 cup of fruit juice added to a quart of water is good. Hydrate throughout your physical activity regimen.

Recommendations for Fluid Before and During Exercise

Time to Drink	Amounts of fluid
2 hours before exercise	1 quart + 1 cup (not all at once)
During exercise (60 to 90 min.)	About 1 quart
After exercise	2 cups fluid for every pound lost

Source: Whitney, E. N., & Sienkiewicz Sizer, F. (1991). *Nutrition Concepts & Controversies, 5th edition.* St. Paul, MN: West Publishing Company.

Supplements for Performance

Increasing physical performance and stamina is sometimes grueling. The bottom line is nothing really takes the place of time and sweat. There are no miracle drugs to make it happen. Before using supplements, read about the pros and cons from credible sources.

Also always let your physician know about all supplements you are using. Review the chart on page 84 regarding some popular supplements taken for enhancing performance (see Resources for more information).

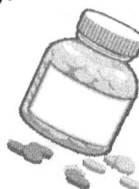

Supplement	Pros	Cons
Beta-Alanine	It _may_ reduce that burning sensation felt during intense exercise	It may interact with some heart medications and drugs taken for erectile dysfunction. Its safety has not been established for people with particular diseases.
Branched Chain Amino Acids	Not harmful, they may work but you won't see dramatic results	Best to take protein as a whole nutrient vs. its broken down constituents such as amino acids
Creatine	Possibly beneficial with short bouts of intense exercise	Taking high doses could cause liver, kidney, or heart damage
Whey Protein	If taken shortly after exercise may reduce muscle damage, however, eating a high protein meal will get these results too	Avoid if you have milk allergy, may cause abnormal heart rhythms, changes in cholesterol levels, increased diabetes risk, increased osteoporosis risk

Here's the Deal!

Exercise or any physical activity is an essential part of total wellness. You must gradually increase your momentum and fuel your body with the nutrients it needs. Start slowly if you have been inactive. Injury usually occurs because you try too much too soon or you do a particular exercise incorrectly.

Be especially particular with your back and knees. More strain is felt in those areas. Get the necessary shoes and wear comfortable clothing when you exercise. If you are in your office remove tight belts, ties or anything that could cause your movements to be constricted.

If you have a packed schedule break up your routine into segments. Exercising for 15 minutes twice daily also improves your physical conditioning. Your body is a machine that needs to be treated with care and personal attention. Tune up your machine and it will soar through life. No supplement can do that for you. Good nutrition and sensible exercise goes a long way.

Your Next Step: Longevity

Notes and Action:

_____

_____

_____

_____

_____

_____

_____

_____

_____

_____

_____

_____

_____

_____

_____

_____

ARMY WELL

Fitness includes
strengthening, toning, and
endurance exercises.

Step 7: Longevity

You know you won't live forever but you will sure die trying. I have included some aspects of studies done on groups of people that seem to have the keys to living longer along with my personal perspectives after spending my entire professional career studying health and wellness topics.

Here are 5 basic keys to longevity:

1. Relationships
2. Physical Activity
3. Nutrition
4. Toxic Waste
5. Purposeful Life

Let's look more closely at each key so that you will be able to make personal adjustments and write your action plan to not only live longer but live a much more fulfilled life.

Relationships

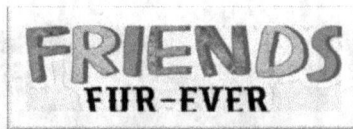

FRIENDS FUR-EVER

I begin this section with one of the most important keys to longevity and that is a good relationship. If you have **one** friend that you trust and who accepts you as you are, then you have found pure gold. More researchers have discovered this essential element to longevity and that is a good quality relationship.

We are made to love and share with one another. John Robbins states in his book, *Healthy at 100,* that the most important indicator of longevity is the quality of our personal relationships and chronic loneliness ranks as one of the most lethal risk factors in determining premature mortality.

Although I am no poet and only have a marginal interest in this area, I thought it was befitting to display the famous poem written by John Donne. "No Man is an Island."

No Man is an Island

No man is an island,
Entire of itself,
Every man is a piece of the continent,
A part of the main.
If a clod be washed away by the sea,
Europe is the less.
As well as if a promontory were.
As well as if a manor of thy friend's
Or of thine own were:
Any man's death diminishes me,
Because I am involved in mankind,
And therefore never send to know for whom
the bell tolls;
It tolls for thee.

Mankind does not live in isolation but our joys, sorrows and hardships are often lessened or enhanced because of our ties to others. When you have friends and family to share your life experiences your joy is increased and your pain diminished.

Develop meaningful friendships with people that are going places and doing positive things. Appreciate your true friends and display your affections through kind words and acts.

Physical Activity

Regular physical activity fuels your mind and body through enhanced circulation. Low intensity physical activity, such as walking is associated with longer life expectancy regardless of body weight, according to a study by a team of researchers led by the National Cancer Institute.

Engaging in leisure-time physical activity can increase your life expectancy as much as 4.5 years. Almost 5 more years added to your life is worth it! This is very important for military operating in low physical active operations.

Nutrition

Nutrition is a science of how your body handles the foods you eat, digest, metabolize, absorb and excrete. In order to function properly and be energized, you need all six nutrients (carbohydrates, proteins, fats, vitamins, minerals, and water).

Carbohydrates

Carbohydrates are the basic fuel for your body. It provides the glucose that enters each cell and keeps it going. Cells in your brain, organs, nails, eyes, etc. are fed through this important nutrient. They supply energy.

Food Sources:

oats, corn, brown rice, quinoa, barley, whole wheat, fruit, vegetables, legumes, pasta, bread, cereal, tortilla

Fats

Fats provide insulation, energy, give structure to cells, provide material for hormonal regulators and carry fat-soluble vitamins in your body.

Food sources:

mayonnaise, salad dressings, oil, gravy, rich sauces, butter, margarine, meat, dairy products, whole grains, nuts, seeds

Proteins

Proteins provide energy, support growth and repair of tissues, help with fluid regulation and acid-base balance. Vital substances such as hormones and enzymes are made from proteins.

Food sources:

nuts, seeds, legumes, lentils, peas, whole grains, tofu, dairy products, quinoa, meats

Vitamins
Organic compounds necessary for vital bodily functions. There are two major categories: water-soluble (B-vitamins, folate, pantothenic acid, biotin and Vitamin C) and fat-soluble (Vitamins A, D, E and K) Food sources: plentiful in all fruits, vegetables, nuts, whole grains, seeds, tofu, meats (eating a wide variety of food is best)
Minerals
Inorganic compounds (chemical elements) necessary for vital bodily functions. There are two categories: major minerals (calcium, chloride, magnesium, phosphorus, potassium, sodium, sulfur) and trace minerals (arsenic, boron, chromium, cobalt, copper, fluoride, iodine, iron, manganese, molybdenum, nickel, selenium, silicon, zinc). Food sources: plentiful in all fruits, vegetables, nuts, whole grains, seeds, tofu, meats (eating a wide variety of food is best)
Water
Water is the river that carries the good substances to the cells and takes away waste products. Functions also include body temperature control, chemical reactions that take place in your body, lubrication and being a shock absorber such as amniotic fluid.

Establish a habit of eating for life. You chose the foods you eat for taste, convenience, economy, culture, habit, or just plain availability. Focus and familiarize yourself with the body's basic nutritional needs if you want to enhance your performance and increase your chances for longevity. A good diet is a strong health defense.

Choose all six nutrients to support growth, maintenance and bodily repair. Just like a car needs gasoline you must have them all to operate efficiently. Also, choose a diet rich in antioxidants. Antioxidants are substances that may protect your cells against free radicals.

Free radicals are produced when you digest food, or by environmental exposures like tobacco smoke and radiation. They can damage cells and may play a role in heart disease, cancer, and other diseases. Chronic and debilitating diseases can often shorten your life expectancy.

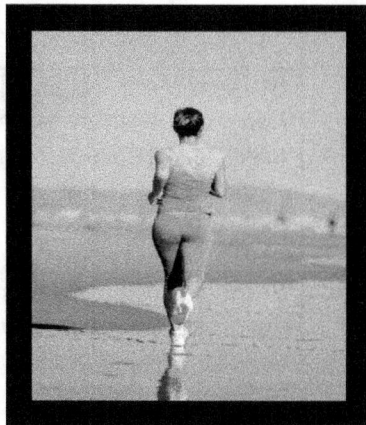

Antioxidant Substance	Food Source
Beta-carotene	Carrots, sweet potato, spinach, dark green leafy vegetables, broccoli, apricot, pumpkin, cantaloupe, mango, squash
Lutein	Spinach, dark green leafy vegetables, broccoli, Brussels sprout, zucchini
Lycopene	Tomatoes, pink grapefruit, watermelon, guava, persimmon, apricots
Selenium	Brazil nuts, brown rice, whole wheat bread, baked beans, Puffed Wheat cereal (fortified), frozen spinach, oatmeal, lentils
Vitamin A	Carrot, tomato, mango, watermelon, peach, sweet potato, pumpkin, zucchini, cantaloupe, dark green leafy vegetables, mandarin orange
Vitamin C	Strawberries, broccoli, potato, kiwi, citrus fruit, parsley, mandarin orange, red/green peppers, cauliflower, mustard greens, pineapple
Vitamin E	Spinach, turnip greens, wheat germ, almond, sunflower seeds, collard greens, peanuts, vegetable oils, broccoli

Also, following a nutrient-rich diet that is low in fat, cholesterol, sodium, and sugar can assist in achieving a healthy weight. Many food products that are not nutrient-dense are high in calories, which can lead to obesity. Being a healthy weight is associated with longer life expectancy.

It's a balancing act that consists of total calories consumed versus total calories expended. Carefully review the calorie content of the foods you choose. If they are high in calories, choose smaller portions or eat them less often. Enjoy your meals but be wise about your frequent selections. You need a diet that supplies you fuel to maintain wellness and a healthy weight.

Diet 101

You get all excited and follow the diet plan to the "t". Usually you lose some weight in the beginning and then start to taper off and eventually fall back to your normal eating patterns. You start to gain much of the weight back and then come across another ritual, and the whole cycle repeats itself.

In the military you have physical guidelines that must be met, and the pressure to be in shape makes following any diet or routine that more difficult. According to one report, 5,000 military men and women are discharged yearly for not meeting weight standards.

Recently a retired Colonel admitted when he was an active soldier he only got serious about his weight just in time to meet the weight standards. Fortunately for him, he met the standards but as mentioned previously many soldiers are not that lucky and are being discharged from the military. The pressure to maintain a certain body weight is tremendous for soldiers and civilians.

To be successful at weight loss you must be realistic and persistent. You can lose weight on any diet but maintaining weight loss is challenging for many people. Always remember quick weight loss schemes get quick results but not always lasting results.

NEWS Flash!!!

"Patience and persistence gets results"

You must have the mind set to see victory. Weight loss is not an overnight venture. If you need support consider a weight loss program such as Weight Watcher's. They have a good track record, and the plan is reasonable.

Several other diet plans on the market can fit into any one of these few categories which are low carbohydrates (carbs) or high protein; starvation or focus on a specific food like the cabbage diet; or eating ready-prepared foods such as those offered on the Jenny Craig or Nutrisystem plan.

Low Carbohydrate/High Protein

The Dietary Guidelines for Americans recommend that carbohydrates should be 45 to 65 percent of your caloric intake. Based on a 2,000 calorie plan, your carbs would range from 225 to 325 grams daily and not less than 130 grams daily according to the Dietary Reference Intakes.

Some popular diets recommend less than 30 grams daily at the beginning of the plan. A carbohydrate intake of less than 20 grams will induce ketosis. Ketosis occurs when glucose is limited and your body creates another path to fuel you. Ketosis can be dangerous.

Starvation plan

A starvation plan is eliminating or drastically reducing carbohydrates and calories. Unless you are under medical supervision, you should not routinely consume less than 1,200 calories.

Starving yourself is characteristic of anorexia nervosa. Also episodes of starving can lead to binge eating. Frequent binge eating and purging, extreme dieting, excessive physical activity, and anorexia are associated with eating disorders.

According to some references, the occurrence of eating disorders is more prevalent in service members than the civilian population. Trying to meet weight standards could resort to these unhealthy acts.

Ready-prepared food systems

Ready-prepared foods such as those offered on the Nutrisystem plan are growing in popularity. The mission is to help you eat better while taking your food choices away to lessen temptation. This plan definitely works for some people not having to worry about portion sizes, grocery shopping, meal planning and cooking.

However, transitioning from the convenience of using ready-prepared foods makes maintaining any weight loss more challenging. Plans like Nutrisystem definitely have their advantages and disadvantages. I know it didn't work for my friend Birchwood who lined the curio cabinet with them. I guess they were just too expensive to toss.

Ponder the following questions for any diet plan you are considering:

Questions?????	
Is the diet plan safe?	Can you continue this plan forever?
Is it satisfying?	How serious are you about changing your lifestyle?
Do you have anyone in your circle of support that can motivate you?	Are your closest associates practicing healthy eating and exercising regularly?

Bottom Line on Popular Diet Plans

Low Carbohydrate/High Protein

You need carbohydrates to increase endurance performance for strenuous training, missions and mental clarity.

Once carbs are digested they supply the fuel as glucose.

Starvation Plan

Drastically limiting calories reduces the fuel and nutrients your body needs for top performance.

Do not follow any plan <1,200 calories unless under medical supervision.

Ready-Prepared Food Systems

The mission is to eat these prepared meals to take the temptation away from making your own food choices. Weaning off the plan and selecting your own foods can be challenging.

For more in-depth guidance contact any resource below:

Online Resources

- **National Eating Disorders Association**: www.edap.org - or call their helpline: 800-931-2237

- **National Institute of Mental Health**, Reducing the burden of mental illness and behavioral disorders through research on mind, brain, and behavior www.nimh.nih.gov

- **National Association of Anorexia Nervosa and Associated Disorders** www.anad.org **Hotline:** 847-831-343, Someone will be able to assist you Monday thru Friday from 9:00 a.m. until 5:00 p.m. CST.

	Men	Women
Body Mass Index (used to determine body fatness)	<40	<35
Waist Circumference measured in centimeters(cm)	<94 cm	<80 cm
Recommended calories for weight loss	1,500 - 1,800	1,200 - 1,500

Always remember the ritual you followed to lose the weight must be maintained. Toss any unsafe dietary plan or regimen that you cannot follow forever. When you are ready to give up the crazy life in the fat lane, here are some practical tips to help you lose sensibly:

1. Try to eat your largest meal at breakfast or noon.

2. Eat late and you'll gain weight

   Note: Night Eating Syndrome is eating excessively in the evening. This disorder is associated with distress and dysfunction. It is prevalent among overweight and obese people.

3. Watch your portions. Take time to measure some of the foods you eat regularly. Read the food labels to ascertain calories. If the calories for a food you choose is 100 calories per serving and the serving size is ½ cup, are you mentally adding the extra 200 calories if your serving is 1 ½ cups?

4. Drink water freely. Sometimes you crave salty and sweet foods when your body actually yearns for water.

5. Be careful of snacking throughout the day. It may be a snack but if you are doing this all day long it packs on the pounds.

6. Note your choice of beverages. Many popular drinks are loaded with calories. Most beverages are 12 – 40 ounces and 8 ounces is a cup.

7. Try a club soda (no calories or sodium) and mix it with some fruit juice.

8. Be physically active, 200 – 300 minutes weekly is associated with weight loss.

Weight gain

Gaining weight is just as tough as losing for some people, particularly service members who must accomplish rigorous physical activities. Guys particularly desire a more hefty or stocky appearance.

I have a soft spot for those who want to gain weight because my dear nephew Carlos had that problem. He would wear big sweat suits and huge coats to make him appear larger.

In the morning he would get on the scale only to realize that he had lost a few pounds just overnight. What a true dilemma for a naturally svelte guy who wanted to gain weight!

Carlos and many other people who have problems gaining weight are probably not consuming enough calories. A real active man may need 3,000 to 4,000 more calories. Just grabbing some food here and there will not suffice. You have to be intentional to add those many calories to your daily plan.

Some quick tips for you to gain weight include the following:

- ✪ Consume three meals daily and healthy snacks.

- ✪ Eat concentrated sources of food such as nutritious smoothies or hot cereals cooked in a nondairy beverage or low fat milk versus plain water.

- ✪ Include at least two healthy snacks such as trail mixes, graham crackers and peanut butter to supplement your meals and don't just "pig out."

- ✪ Try peanut butter and preserves or peanut butter and jam sandwiches.

- ✪ Eat plenty of nutritious high carbohydrate vegetables (yams, sweet potatoes, peas, potatoes) or cream soups.

Try toppings such as coconut shreds, slivered almonds, walnuts, fruit sauces or yogurt.

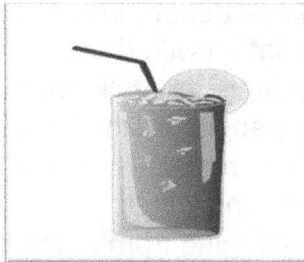

Participating in physical fitness tests and other grueling exercises requires plenty of calories. If you want to gain weight, follow the tips and eat from all food groups.

Toxic Waste

This section on toxic waste and longevity is probably the most important. Toxic waste is material that can cause injury or even death to living creatures. Toxic waste in your life can be negative people, smoking, and unmanaged stress which can all lessen a long productive life.

"Toxic People"

Who are the toxic people in your life? They are the ones who make you feel stupid, angry, disrespected, unworthy or shameful. They are the ones who rob you of your vitality, inner peace and precious time.

Think of your close associates and ask yourself these simple questions:

- ✪ Do these people support my goals and dreams?
- ✪ Am I in a better place because of my association with them?
- ✪ Do they usually talk positively about other people or situations?
- ✪ Do I feel motivated or energized after associating with them?
- ✪ Am I learning from them?

If your answers are primarily no, then you have toxic people in your life. Are most of your close associates lethal? Then <u>you</u> must make a decision to eliminate or lessen your time spent with these individuals. Tactics for handling difficult talks with toxic people are as follows:

✪ Realize that you can only change you.

✪ Be honest about your role in this hostile interaction.

✪ Don't raise the steam by becoming hostile. A softly spoken answer can diffuse the situation.

✪ Be firm in your encounter with someone who becomes disrespectful. Simply say, "I will continue talking when you address me in a more civil manner."

✪ If you must talk further make sure it is at a mutually agreeable time.

✪ Remember your objective is how you feel about the encounter or what you felt led to this ordeal. For example, "I feel my request for leave is often denied because of your personal feelings toward me and not my performance."

✪ Be specific in what you would like to occur between the two of you.

Wherever you go you will meet people who are stuck in the past or who consciously or subconsciously want to pull you down. It is your choice to seek higher ground and to seek more positive associates.

>**Note:** If you cannot dispose of them, then limit and set strict boundaries to your interactions with toxic people. The choice is yours.

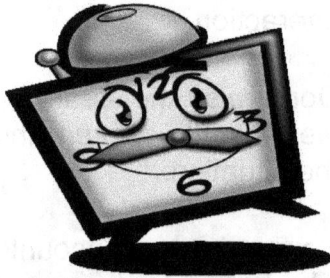

Stress

Unmanaged stress is a toxic waste. Stress negatively impacts your health if not managed well and can take productive years from your life. Experts have associated heart problems, cancer, backaches, and problems focusing or concentrating with stress. Incorporate these five fundamental strategies to manage stress.

Five Stress Strategies

1. Physical activity

Exercise daily and at your own pace to rejuvenate your body and mind.

2. Good nutrition

Eat to nourish your body and adhere to the guidelines outlined in meal planning.

---

3. Relaxation techniques

You will feel more refreshed to take on tasks when you are mentally and physically less stressed. The relationship between the mental and physical state is closely interwoven. An unhealthy mental state can affect your overall health.

Stressors are compounded for those in the military. Practice easy relaxation techniques. Sit in a comfortable chair with good back support. Try tensing muscle groups for ten seconds and then relaxing them. Start with your face, neck, shoulders, hands, buttocks, thighs, calves and then toes. Do these techniques two or three times.

Also put a cool wet cloth on your forehead of the back of your neck. Sit quietly in a comfortable chair and just let go.

While relaxing, choose music that creates a calm atmosphere. Listening to classical music especially releases stress and increases clarity of thought, according to Dr. Neil Nedley (a full-time practicing physician in Internal Medicine emphasizing Lifestyle Medicine, Mental Health, and Depression Recovery).

Most people must acquire a taste for classical music. You may prefer classic rock, top 40's, country, hip hop or contemporary blues; however, easy classical music soothes your soul.

---

4. Task management

A pile of tasks and deadlines causes stress and impacts quality sleep. Adjust tasks to what you can successfully manage. We all possess varying aptitudes and skills. As soon as your duty is assigned start filing it by using three categories (Due Today, Due in 2-days, By the end of the week). Focus on the most important task for that day. This requires discipline.

Due Today: (an example)

Task #1 (target completion – by 9:00 a.m.)

Task #2 (target completion – by 1:30 p.m.)

Task #3 (target completion - by 3:45 p.m.)

I start with a complete understanding of the entire task and then I break it up into smaller segments and set deadlines for each activity. I always allow a little room for interruptions or for those days when you just need a break.

108

Most procrastinators want to do a good job, but get so overwhelmed with the task and delay getting started. Taking small steps makes larger jobs more manageable. I always use this technique, even to write this book, which my editor is patiently awaiting to review.

Make sure to take several breaks so you won't be so overwhelmed with the project at hand. I also try to do the worst part of the project first to get it out of the way.

---

5. Assertiveness techniques

Using assertiveness techniques helps you to clearly express your legitimate rights, communicate more effectively, and release stress. Oftentimes people try to bully, manipulate or intimidate you with their caustic words. By letting others know your boundaries, sets the tone for open discussions and mutual respect. You earn respect, it is not always automatically granted.

Purposeful Life

You have chosen to serve your country. What an awesome career choice! Your decision to serve is just the beginning. As you continue to grow and achieve, you must still decide your purpose in life. This is your life.

What do you enjoy doing? What makes you feel satisfied deep inside? What are your dreams and passions? What specific service can you bring to mankind to make a decided difference? When you know the answers to these questions you can begin to embark on a purposeful life. You will achieve. You will grow.

"If you fail to plan, then you plan to fail" –
Harvey Mackay

Harvey Mackay is a businessman and columnist. He is also the author of five bestsellers and a popular public speaker.

Note: Learn from someone who has achieved a purposeful life.

A day without a plan is as if you are trying to shoot a target in the dark. I was told success comes before work only in the dictionary. An effective approach to success is setting precise daily goals. Don't worry about how you will achieve the goals. Money, tools, technology or whatever are not the focus when you write your goals. Those things will be addressed later.

Start by determining your long-term goals. Long-terms goals are your desires or dreams you wish to accomplish in the next three to five years. Usually people set goals based on their current skills or interests. You may need to acquire some skills to pursue your goals.

Note: Use your natural abilities

Warren Buffet a billionaire likes numbers. He has a photographic memory as well. These natural abilities, plus what he was willing to <u>learn</u> from the experts, made him rich, rich, rich and richer. Mr. Buffet admits he doesn't know a whole lot about technical things. Fortunately for him, he can pay someone else to address those areas he lacks. He greatly enjoys what he does using his natural abilities, and he is willing to work hard.

My good friend Rob wanted to be a Navy SEAL but he wasn't a strong enough swimmer. Subsequently, he decided to join the Army and is now retired managing several businesses. Sometimes you don't realize your ultimate dream, but at least make an attempt before you quit. Follow these 5 rules for accomplishing your dreams and purposeful life:

Make a list

Long-term goals

Short-term goals

Objectives

Address obstacles

Rule #1 – Make a list

Decide what you want to accomplish. Make a list of the things you enjoy doing in your pastime. Try not to intellectualize this activity and just jot down what comes to mind.

Rule #2 – Long-term goals

Goals are those broad desires you want to achieve. These are general statements of your aspirations. You don't have to be specific while writing goals. These are the goals you want to accomplish in three to five years.

Rule #3 – Short-term goals

Short-term goals can be achieved usually within a year and could be the steps toward your long-term goals or they could be totally different.

Long-term goals (examples)
✪ Train soldiers and their families on the 8 Steps to Total Wellness. ✪ I will graduate with a degree in computer science.
Short-term goals (examples)
✪ Write the 8 Steps to Total Wellness book. ✪ I will enroll in a computer science class this semester.

Rule #4 – Objectives

Objectives are the specific actions needed to actualize your goals. They should be measurable and easily determined. Write awesome objectives by including the action (see Action Words) to be accomplished, level of attainment, and the completion time.

Your road to a purposeful life must be structured. By writing detailed objectives you can measure your success along the way.

Action Words
Accomplish, Achieve, Assess, Build, Buy, Cancel, Create, Correct, Cost, Decide, Develop, Fix, Generate, Graduate, Manage, Prepare, Register, Schedule, Select, Show, Specify, State, Summarize, Translate
Example of objectives (measurable)
✪ I will achieve an 80% or better average by midterm in the computer science class. (action – I will achieve) (level of attainment – 80% or better average) (time period – by midterm of that semester)

> ✪ I will save $300.00 needed to purchase all materials recommended for the computer science class before the fall semester.
>
> (action – I will save $$$)
> (level of attainment - $300.00)
> (time period – before the fall semester)
>
> ✪ I will select a professional cover for the book 8 Steps to Total Wellness by the end of the month.
>
> (action – I will select a book cover)
> (level of attainment – a <u>professional</u> book cover)
> (time period – by the end of the month)

Your objectives must relate to your specific goals and be easily evaluated or measured. They are the rungs on the ladder leading to the accomplishment of your goals. Always include the level of achievement, the designated time frame, and the targeted action.

Note: Your written goals and objectives are the keys to planning your purposeful life.

Rule #5 - Address obstacles

Now the hard part is to get moving. You have to really decide what is holding you back or what are your obstacles.

Identify those obstacles and then write an action plan to overcome them. I have written an example of addressing some of the obstacles for publishing and distributing the book - ARMY WELL - 8 Steps to Total Wellness. After you write a book there are many steps before it gets to the bookstore or on amazon.com. There are several hurdles and challenges to overcome.

ARMY WELL - Addressing Obstacles

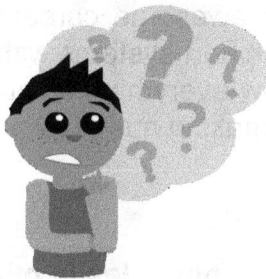

How will I finance publishing?

How will I get my book distributed?

- ✪ Get a loan
- ✪ Get a part time job to earn more $$$
- ✪ Use money from savings accout
- ✪ Get my friend Birchwood to assist with distribution
- ✪ Select publisher
- ✪ Register with amazon.com

Outline your plan and get help if you need it. What resources do you need? Ask others who have accomplished similar goals to give you credible resources to help you move forward.

Don't be too concerned about not having all the facts or an exact plan of how to accomplish your goals.

I included this section on longevity to help you with foundational areas of life that impact achieving quality living. It is a complex wheel that includes careful planning and your per-sistence in following.

You have this awesome career in the military and several support systems within your reach. You won't know everything all at once. You will grow through making mistakes and experience.

Keep these five pinciples in mind as you continue to grow:

1. Select healthy relationships
2. Choose good nutrition
3. Participate in regular physical activity
4. Dispose of toxic waste
5. Plan your long purposeful life

Here's the Deal!

You pack your own suitcase. If you don't have a toothbrush, pajamas, comb, or a book to read, it's on you. You packed it. I understand that some of you will have much harder challenges to overcome. See those hardships as your tools being sharpened. To get to the top you have to climb. A successful life does not have to be equated with how much money you make or how many letters you have after your name. But it does mean that you truly have dreams that are deeply embedded and your life would be much more fulfilled living those dreams.

Remember success comes before work only in the dictionary. Anticipate difficulties, disappointments, delays, and rejection. It prepares you for the road ahead. No one really remembers how many times they fell off their bike when they first learned to ride. You do however remember the joy of riding.

Total wellness is a journey worth pursuing. You pack your own suitcase. Learn the steps and incorporate them diligently into your purposeful life. It's your time!

Your Next Step: Leisure

Notes and Action:

_____

_____

_____

_____

_____

_____

_____

_____

_____

_____

_____

_____

_____

_____

_____

ARMY WELL

Your days are numbered;
live every day to the
fullest.

Step 8: Leisure

Nothing can restore and rejuvenate your body more than leisure time. Can you imagine no schedule, duty, business, chores, or commitments to meet? You spend this time living in the moment. Leisure is the true reward to a disciplined existence.

If your brain is weary and your nerves on edge, then take a drive to the country and surround yourself in nature. Stroll through the fields and woods stopping to pick wild flowers or watch the butterflies. Being near nature is the best remedy for your weary soul.

To stay in the wellness zone the leisure time spent must be uplifting. True recreation refreshes your mind and body. Leisure activities can be physical or sedentary.

Hearing the ocean waves, feeling the crisp breeze, smelling the salt water, or viewing a sea gull travel the horizon all capture pure leisurely moments.

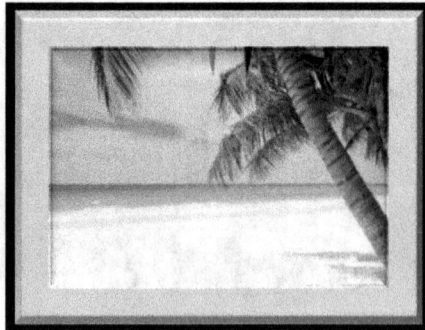

I was at a private beach my last vacation. Hearing the ocean waves and also watching the sea creatures just did wonders for me like no other activity. I sat in the sand right on the beach and allowed the waves to splash me.

What an adventure when I saw both a stingray and a shark! It was a small shark, and I was completely captivated at its swift movement through the water.

Leisure activities don't always have to be expensive. I make a point to do a pleasurable pastime at least once a week. Some of these outings cost money and others are little or no cost. Sometimes I want to venture alone, and other times I include family and friends.

The most interesting people I know live by indulging in their hobbies and not just watching others participate. Choose to get in the game and don't be just a spectator.

What are your hobbies or fun activities? How often do you engage in recreation? Remember when you participate in true recreation you leave feeling refreshed or inspired.

Watching an intense horror movie would not constitute as being uplifting or refreshing. Painting, creative writing, woodworking, sailing, hiking, camping, drawing, cooking, skating, and bicycling are all invigorating pastimes.

What are your excuses for delaying enjoyment? Are you too busy for leisure? Oftentimes after true recreation, you are more productive. The point is to make this happen for you. Make your list of fun things you want to do and do them.

High achievers like both Spencer Rascoff and Larnelle Harris engage regularly in leisure activities. Mr. Rascoff co-founded Hotwire.com and served as Vice President for Expedia and Chief Executive Officer at Zillow. According to this CEO, his weekends are an important time to unplug from the day-to-day. He always spends time with his family.

Larnelle Harris is a famous gospel singer who won five Grammy awards,18 Dove awards and achieved several number one songs on the inspirational music charts. Regardless of his hectic schedule, Mr. Harris insists on being home on the weekends with his family and being involved with his church.

> **Note:** If these over-achievers can find some downtime, then I know you can also. It is the foundation of a total wellness plan called balance. Leisure is not a luxury it is a necessity.

Engaging in recreational activities, particularly outdoors, definitely improves your physical wellness. According to Dr. Laura Payne of the University of Illinois, people who visited the park had fewer doctor visits, lower body mass indexes and lower systolic blood pressures than those who didn't. Moreover, you get fresh oxygen, and a natural source of Vitamin D from the sunshine.

When I was growing up I would hear the saying, "all work and no play makes Jack a dull boy." In other words, add spice to your life. Come out of your shell and expand your horizons. You don't need to be a millionaire to enjoy life. The most wonderful joys are free. All you need is to schedule the time and an openness to let go and engage yourself.

Frequently choose activities that truly rejuvenate and add zest to your life. You gain more coping power by balancing the stresses of life with pure leisure.

Here's the Deal!

Make leisure activities a priority. According to your schedule or assignment, you may have to include short periods of downtime. You need the balance from mental anguish, deadlines, projects, competitions or just routine.

In addition, be creative if you do not have the tools or resources to do everything you want to do. Kids are great at making things happen with little or nothing.

The saddest story begins with "I wish I had done...." Leisure activities do not have to be expensive or in some far away country. Review your list and participate in those hobbies or interests you listed.

You pack your own suitcase so make sure you make room for sheer enjoyment. It's your time and you are worth it. Start today with the last but not least step of ⇒⇒⇒⇒⇒⇒⇒⇒

ARMY WELL - 8 Steps to Total Wellness.

Notes and Action:

ARMY WELL

The years are what you make them; let your years be long and wonderful!!!

Practice Exercise II

The answers to these questions are in Appendix C.

1. List the 5 basic keys to longevity.

2. Oranges, apples, meats and dairy are significant sources of beta-carotene. (True or False)

3. Adults need 1.5 milliliters of fluid per kilocalorie. (True or False)

4. Which type of water is high in sodium?
   a. Fluoridated   c. Distilled
   b. Pure Water   d. Mineral

5. Exercising even 15 minutes twice daily also improves your physical conditioning. (True or False)

6. People who engaged in physical activity during their leisure time had life expectancy gains of as much as 4.5 years. (True or False)

7. I will graduate with a degree in social work is an example of a long-term goal. (True or False)

8. All types of music that you like can release stress. (True or False)

9. Chronic loneliness is associated with premature mortality. (True or False)

10. The Dietary Guidelines for Americans recommend a carbohydrate intake of 20 grams daily. (True or False)

SUMMARY

Your fitness challenge requires your full participation. This is not a dream or merely a thought process. The more input, the more output. Eight steps are incorporated (air, rest, meal planning, yield, water, exercise, longevity, and leisure) to increase your fitness factor.

Accept the consequences of your actions or lack of them. Take one step at a time. Practice that one behavior until it becomes your routine. Embrace it, breath it, feel it, and definitely do it. Make the decision today to move in a more positive and healthier direction.

Spend your life feeling good, looking good, and lengthening your days. Learn from previous failed attempts and move forward and take the next step.

Try to understand what really caused the problem. Were you realistic in your endeavors? Carefully review your previous failed attempts and make the necessary adjustments.

All eight steps are needed to achieve optimal health and wellness. You read the material, now it's time to come out of the laboratory and execute.

Remember:

You're not well unless you're
ARMY WELL

━━━━━━━━━━━━━━━━━━━━

We thank our dedicated service members who
have and are leading, guarding, meeting,
strategizing, and tirelessly fighting for our
freedom. Your sacrifices cannot be measured.
We especially want you to be ARMY STRONG
and capture the medal of total wellness.

APPENDICES

Appendix A – I. Meal Planning

Meal Planning Template – Use all food groups, write your menu, and make sure you include adequate daily servings.

Dairy/Non-Dairy 2 - 3 servings	Fruit/Veg 5 - 13 servings	Protein 2 servings	Grain 6 – 8 ounces
Breakfast			
Lunch			
Dinner			
Snack			

II. Meal Planning Reservoir

Use this guide to ensure a wide variety of food selections when meal planning.

Protein Group	Protein (no meat)
Alfredo Chicken	Bean Burgers*
Baked Chicken	Bean Burrito
Baked Fish	Beans N' Rice
BBQ Chicken	Big D's Meatloaf**
Beef Patties	Black Bean Mexicana*
Beef Tips	Black Bean Soup*
Braised Beef	Black-eyed Peas*
Breaded Fish	Eggs
Chicken Salad	E-Zee Chicken Salad***
Chicken Strips	Falafel
Chicken Teriyaki	Garden Burger
Chili	Italian Meatballs*
Lasagna	Lentils*(*Lentil Stew*)
Meatloaf	Macaroni N' Cheese**
Roast Turkey	(featured in *Real Health*
Sloppy Jo	*Magazine*)
Spaghetti & Meatsauce	Nuts
Steak	Savory Nuggets***
Tunafish	Sloppy Jo***
Turkey Casserole	Spaghetti & Tomato Sauce
Turkey N' Noodles	Seeds
Turkey N' Gravy	Split Peas*
	Textured Vegetable
	Protein or Meat
	Substitutes
	Tofu*(Pa's Sunrise
	Scrambles)
	Veggie Chili*
	Veggie Lasagna

Dairy Group	Non Dairy Group

Evaporated Skim
Frozen Yogurt
Fruit Yogurt
Low fat 2% Milk
Low fat Buttermilk
Low fat Ice Cream
Plain Nonfat Yogurt
Skim Milk
Whole Milk
 	
The choices underlined add more calories due to the extra sugar. Ice cream contains more fat and sugar.
	Almonds ¼ cup
	Blackstrap Molasses
	Fortified Almond
	  Milk
	Fortified Coconut
	  Milk
	Fortified Rice milk
	Fortified Soymilk
	Fortified Soymilk
	  Products (pudding,
	  ice cream)
	Tofu (processed
	  with calcium)

Grains	Fruits
Barley Bulgur Brown Rice Buckwheat Corn Couscous Graham Millet Oatmeal Triticale Rye Whole Wheat	Apple Avocado Banana Blueberries Cherries Kiwi Grapefruit Grapes Lemon Mango Orange Peach Pear Pineapple Plum Raisins Strawberries Tangerine Watermelon

Vegetables	Note:
Acorn Squash Beets Bok Choy Broccoli Brussels Sprout Cabbage Carrots Cauliflower Celery Collards Corn Green Beans Green Peas Kale Mustard Grens Okra Parsnips Potatoes Pumpkin Spinach Sweet Potatoes Turnips Yams Zucchini	The Meal Planning Reservoir is used to help you provide a wider variety of meals. Sometimes we get into a rut and fix the same foods. Explore different proteins, fruits, grains and vegetables. A wide variety of food selections also helps to ensure you are getting the nutrients you need. No one food provides everything and that is why you must plan your meals using all of the food groups. Experiment, have fun, and enjoy your meals!

For additional meal plans see http://myplate.gov/

* Smith, Donna A. *Pumpkin's Veggie Delights*. Madison: Health Opera Press, 1998.
**Smith, Donna A. *Whole Food Soul Food – Finger Lickin' Way to Fight the Fat.* 2003.
***Smith, Donna A. *Finger Lickin' Way to Fight the Fat.* Bangor: Booklocker, 2005.

2000 Calorie Meal	Sample Menu
Breakfast No. of Choices: 1 Milk 1 Fruit 2 Bread/Starch 1 Meat/Meat Alternate 2 Fat	1 cup Soymilk 1 Apple 2 Slices Whole Grain Toast 1 Egg (Egg Substitute) or Pa's Sunrise Scrambles** 2 teaspoons Margarine

Lunch
No. of Choices:
0 Milk
1 Vegetable
1 Fruit
2 Bread/Starch
2 Meat/Meat Alternate
1 Fat
	Garden Salad with fat-free
	   Salad Dressing
	1 Pear
	2 Slices Whole Grain
	   Bread
	2 oz. Baked Chicken Patty
	   or Lentil Burger*
	1 teaspoon Mayonnaise

Mid Afternoon Snack No. of Choices: 1 Bread/starch 1 Meat/Meat Alternate	6 Whole Grain Crackers 2 tablespoons Peanut Butter

Dinner
No. of Choices:
1 Milk/Milk Alternate
2 Vegetable
1 Fruit
2 Bread/Starch
2 Meat/Meat Alternate
1 Fat
	1 Serving Fortified Soy
	   Pudding
	1 cup Green Beans
	½ cup Natural Applesauce
	⅓ cup Brown Rice
	1 Whole Grain Dinner
	   Rolls
	2 oz. Italian Meatballs*
	1 teaspoon Margarine

* Smith, Donna A. *Pumpkin's Veggie Delights*. Madison: Health Opera Press, 1998.
**Smith, Donna A. *Whole Food Soul Food – Finger Lickin' Way to Fight the Fat*. Mckinney: Magni Publishing, 2003.

III. Seasonal Food Purchasing

Use this guide for buying seasonal fresh fruits and vegetables. You get better quality and save money when you buy in seson.

January/February	
Fruits	*Vegetables*
Apple	Artichokes(Feb.)
Avocado	Beets
Grapefruit	Cabbage
Lemons	Cauliflower
Navel orange	Celery
Tangerine	Lettuce
Winter pear	Potato
	Spinach
March/April	
Apple	Artichoke
Avocados	Beets
Grapefruit	Broccoli
Lemon	Cabbage
Navel orange	Carrot
Strawberries(April)	Cauliflower
Winter pear	Celery(March)
	Lettuce(April)
	Peas(April)
	Potato
	Spinach(April)

May/June	
Apricot(June)	Beet(May)
Avocado	Cabbage(May)
Bush berries(June)	Carrots
Cantaloupe(June)	Celery
Cherries	Cucumber(June)
Grapefruit(May)	Green beans(June)
Honeydew melon(June)	Lettuce
Lemon	Onion
Orange	Peas(May)
Nectarine(June)	Pepper(June)
Peach(June)	Potato
Plum(June)	Spinach(May)
Strawberries(June)	Squash(June)
Watermelon(June)	Sweet corn
	Tomato

July/August	
Apricot(July)	Cabbage
Avocado	Carrots
Bush berries(July)	Celery
Cantaloupe	Cucumber
Grapefruit	Eggplant
Honeydew melon	Green beans
Lemon	Lettuce
Nectarine	Onion
Orange	Pepper
Peach	Potato
Plum	Squash
Strawberries(July)	Sweet corn
Watermelon	Tomato

137

September/October	
Fruits	Vegetables
Apple	Broccoli(Oct.)
Cantaloupe(Sept.)	Cabbage
Grapefruit(Sept.)	Cucumber
Grapes	Green beans
Honeydew melon(Sept.)	Lettuce(Oct.)
Lemon	Lima beans(Oct.)
Orange(Oct.)	Onion
Peach(Sept.)	Peas
Pear	Potato(Oct.)
Plum(Oct.)	Squash
Prune(Oct.)	Sweet corn
	Sweet potato(Oct.)
	Tomato
November/December	
Apple	Broccoli
Avocado	Carrot(Dec.)
Grapefruit(Dec.)	Cauliflower(Dec.)
Grapes(Nov.)	Celery(Dec.)
Lemon	Lettuce(Nov.)
Orange(Dec.)	Potato(Dec.)
Walnuts	Spinach(Dec.)
	Squash(Dec.)
	Sweet potato(Dec.)

Note: "Use by" or "sell by" date lets the store manager know how long to display a food product; after this date the food quality or taste diminishes. Don't buy or eat food after the expiration date. It could be on the verge of spoiling.

Appendix B – Practice I.

These are the answers to Practice I.

1.   For this exercise you must write what you ate for a day and compare your results to the recommended daily food groups.

Breakfast	Lunch
1 cup Orange Juice 1 cup of Corn Flakes 1 cup of Milk	Hamburger(3 oz.) 1 Donut
Dinner	
Baked Fish (3 ounces) ½ Mixed Vegetables 1 Slice Whole Wheat Bread 12 ounce Soda	

Food Groups	Daily Recommended
Dairy	2 to 3 servings/2 to 3 cups
Protein	2 servings/5 -6 ounces
Fruits/Veg.	5 – 13 servings/2 ½ to 6 ½ Cups
Grains	6 to 8 ounces

Actual Amounts Eaten - Sample Meal Comparison of Daily Recommended Food Groups
Dairy = 1 cup Protein = 6 ounces Fruits/Vegetables = 1 ½ cups Grains = 4 ounces

Summary: In this meal you must add more dairy choices, fruits/vegetables and grains to meet the daily recommendations.

2. Rapid Eye Movement (REM) and Non Rapid Eye Movement (NREM).
3. False
4. a. Water, fat and protein
5. True
6. True
7. a. Potato chips, stick margarine, partially hydrogenated fats
8. True
9. 400 milligrams
10. True

Appendix C – Practice II

These are the answers to Practice II. Also for additional credible information refer to the Resource section of this book.

1. Relationships, physical activity, nutrition, toxic waste and a purposeful life
2. False
3. True
4. Mineral
5. True
6. True
7. True
8. False
9. True
10. False

RESOURCES

Physical Activity Plan:

1. http://health.state.ga.us/pdfs/family
   health/nutrition/

2. http://www.mayoclinic.com/health/fitness
   /MY00396

Nutritional data:

1. Smith, Donna A. *Pumpkin's Veggie Delights*. Madison: Health Opera Press, 1998.
2. Smith, Donna A. *Finger Lickin' Way to Fight the Fat*. Bangor: Booklocker, 2005.
3. Smith, Donna A. *Whole Food Soul Food – Finger Lickin' Way to Fight the Fat*. Mckinney: Magni Publishing, 2003.
4. Smith, Donna A. *The Health Stop Plan*. Madison: Health Opera Press, 2010.
5. www.healthopera.biz
6. http://myplate.gov/
7. http://www.vrg.org
8. http://nat.illinois.edu/
9. http://www.myfoodrecord.com
10. http://www.fns.usda.gov/slp
11. http://ndb.nal.usda.gov/ndb/foods/
12. http://www.eatright.org

REFERENCES

Step 1: Air

White, E. G. (1942) *The Ministry of Healing*, Mountain View, CA: Pacific Press.

"Indoor Air Quality"
Retrieved from-
https://www.osha.gov/SLTC/indoorairquality/

"Stress Management: Breathing Exercises for Relaxation"
Retrieved from-
http://www.webmd.com/balance/stress-management/stress-management-breathing-exercises-for-relaxation

"Efficient Breathing Reduces Health Risks, Including Heart Attacks"
Retrieved from-
http://www.drdavidwilliams.com/proper-breathing-improves-health/

Step 2: Rest

"Sleep and Health"
Retrieved from-
http://healthysleep.med.harvard.edu/need-sleep/whats-in-it-for-you/health

143

Colten HR and Altevogt BM, eds. *Sleep Disorders and Sleep Deprivation: An Unmet Public Health Problem*. Board on Health Sciences Policy; National Academies Press. 2006.

"Definition (Sleep Disorder)"
Retrieved from-
http://www.mayoclinic.org/diseases-conditions/sleep-disorders/ basics/ definition/con-20037263

A resource from the Division of Sleep Medicine at Harvard Medical School Produced in partnership with WGBH Educational Foundation
Retrieved from-
http://healthysleep.med.harvard.edu /need-sleep/whats-in-it-for-you/health

"Role of Sleep Duration and Quality in the Risk and Severity of Type 2 Diabetes Mellitus." Kristen L. Knutson, PhD; Armand M. Ryden, MD; Bryce A. Mander, BA; Eve Van Cauter, PhD *Arch Intern Med.* 2006;166(16):1768-1774.doi:10.1001/ archinte.166.16.1768.

"Sleep Duration and Body Mass Index in a Rural Population." –
Neal D. Kohatsu, MD, MPH; Rebecca Tsai, MS; Terry Young, PhD; Rachel VanGilder, PhD; Leon F. Burmeister, PhD; Ann M. Stromquist, PhD; James A. Merchant, MD, DrPH *Arch Intern Med.* 2006;166(16):1701-1705. doi:10.1001/archinte.166.16.1701.

"Rest"
> Retrieved from-http://newstartclub.com/ resources/detail/rest

Step 3: Meal Planning

Choose My Plate.gov
> Retrieved from- http://myplate.gov/

"Eating Disorders in the Military"
> Retrieved from- http://jama.jamanetwork.com/article.asp x?articleid=1842744

"Eating Disorders High Among Military Women"
> Retrieved from-http://eatingdisorders review.com/nl/nl/_edr_11_2_4.html

Lindquist, C. H., & Bray, R. M. "Trends in overweight and physical activity among U.S. military personnel."1995-1998. *Prev Med.* January 2001; 32(1):57-65.

National Nutrient Database for Standard Reference, Release 26, The National Agricultural Library.

Smith, Donna A. (2005) *Finger Lickin' Way to Fight the Fat.* Bangor: Booklocker.

Child and Adult Care Food Program – Nutrition Guidance for Child Care Homes. United States Department of Agriculture – Food and Consumer Service. September 1995.

"Do Food Expiration Dates Really Matter?"
Retrieved from-
http://www.webmd.com/a-to-z-
guides/features/do-food-expiration-
dates-matter

Step 4: Yield

"Are We Too Sweet? Our Kids' Addiction to Sugar"
Retrieved from-
http://life.familyeducation.com/nutritional
information/obesity/64270.html

"Sugar and Carbohydrates"
Retrieved from-http://www.heart.org/
HEARTORG/GettingHealthy/Nutrition
Center/HealthyDietGoals/Sugars-and-
Carbohydrates_UCM_303296_Article.
jsp

"Sugar Drinks and Obesity Fact Sheet"
Retrieved from-
http://www.hsph.harvard.edu/nutrition
source/sugary-drinks-fact-sheet/

"Potential role of sugar (fructose) in the
epidemic of hypertension, obesity and the
metabolic syndrome, diabetes, kidney disease,
and cardiovascular disease"
Retrieved from-
http://ajcn.nutrition.org/content/86/4/899.
full

"The Truth About Agave"
Retrieved from-http://www.webmd.com/
diet/features/the-truth-about-agave

"Agave: Why We Were Wrong"
Retrieved from-http://blog.doctoroz.com/
dr-oz-blog/agave-why-we-were-wrong

"What Are the Benefits From Coconut Sugar?"
Retrieved from-http://www.livestrong.
com/article/367337-what-are-the-
benefits-of-coconut-sugar/

"10 Artificial Sweeteners and Sugar
Substitutes"
Retrieved from-http://www.health.com/
health/gallery/0,,20424821,00.html

"Chemical Cuisine Learn About Food
Additives"
Retrieved from-
http://www.cspinet.org/reports/chemcuisi
ne.htm#artificialsweeteners

"Infant Botulism"
Retrieved from-
http://kidshealth.org/parent/infections/ba
cterial_viral/botulism.html

"Know Your Fats "
Retrieved from-
http://www.heart.org/HEARTORG/Condi
tions/Cholesterol/PreventionTreatmentof
HighCholesterol/Know-Your-Fats_UCM
_305628_Article.jsp

"High Blood Cholesterol Levels"
        Retrieved from-
        http://www.nlm.nih.gov/medlineplus/enc
        y/article/000403.htm

"Fat Shockers: Surprisingly High-Fat Foods"
        Retrieved from-http://www.webmed.com
        /food-recipes/features/fat-shockers-sur
        prisingly-high-fat-foods

"National Nutrient Database for Standard
Reference"
        Retrieved from-
        http://ndb.nal.usda.gov/ndb/

"The Phantom Fat"
        Retrieved from-https://www.cspinet.
        org/nah/septrans.html

"Arteriosclerosis/atherosclerosis"
        Retrieved from-http://www.mayoclinic.
        org/diseases-conditions/arterioosclero
        sis-atherosclerosis/basics/symptoms/
        con-20026972

"The Truth About 7 Common Food Additives"
        Retrieved from-
        http://www.webmd.com/diet/features/the
        -truth-about-seven-common-food-
        additives?page=3

"Worst Fast Food Meals for Sodium"
        Retrieved from-
        http://www.cnn.com/2013/01/04/health/
        gallery/fast-food-worst-sodium-meals

"What is Propionate?"
    Retrieved from-
    http://www.livestrong.com/article/501045
    -what-is-sodium-propionate/

Whitney, E. N., & Sienkiewicz Sizer, F. (1991).
Nutrition Concepts & Controversies, 5th edition.
St. Paul, MN: West Publishing Company.

"Medicines in my Home: Caffeine in Your
Body"
    Retrieved from-
    http://www.fda.gov/downloads/drugs/res
    ourcesforyou/... the.../ucm205286.pdf

"Caffeine Content of Food and Drugs" –
Center for Science in the Public Interest
    Retrieved from-
    http://www.cspinet.org/new/cafchart.htm

"Caffeine Content of Popular Drinks"
    Retrieved from-http:/www.math.utah.edu
    /~yplee/fun/caffeine.html

"Caffeine: How Much Is Too Much?" By Mayo
Clinic Staff
    Retrieved from-http://www.mayoclinic.
    org/healthy-living/nutrition-and-healthy-
    eating/in-depth/caffeine/art-20045678

Step 5: Water

Whitney, E. N., Cataldo, C. B., & Rolfes, S. R.
(1994). *Understanding Normal & Clinical
Nutrition.* St. Paul, MN: West Publishing
Company.

Step 6: Exercise

Whitney, E. N., & Sienkiewicz Sizer, F. (1991). *Nutrition Concepts & Controversies, 5th edition*. St. Paul, MN: West Publishing Company.

Sharffenberg, J. A., MD, MPH. "Nutrition in Exercise."

"Exercise at Your Desk"
Retrieved from-
http://www.webmd.com/fitness-exercise/features/exercise-at-your-desk

"Avoiding Knee or Hip Surgery"
Retrieved from-
http://www.health.harvard.edu/newsletters/Harvard_Health_Letter/2013/June/avoiding-knee-or-hip-surgery

"Whey Protein"
Retrieved from- http://www.mayoclinic.org/drugs-supplements/whey-protein/safety/hrb-20060532

"Beta-alanine"
Retrieved from-http://www.webmd.com/vitamins-and-supplements/beta-alanine-uses-and-risks#3

"Dementia"
Retrieved from-
http://www.mayoclinic.org/diseases-conditions/dementia/basics/definition/con-20034399

"Do Supplements Give Athletes an Edge?"
Retrieved from-
http://www.webmd.com/vitamins-and-supplements/features/athletic-supplements-fact-fiction?page=2

Step 7: Longevity

"The Surprising Secret to Health and Longevity"
Retrieved from-
http://www.psychologytoday.com/blog/stronger-the-broken-places/201304/the-surprising-secret-health-and-longevity

Smith, Donna A. (2005) *Finger Lickin' Way to Fight the Fat.* Bangor: Booklocker.

"Healthy Diet: Do You Follow Dietary Guidelines?"
Retrieved from-
http://www.mayoclinic.org/healthy-living/nutrition-and-healthy-eating/in-depth/how-to-eat-healthy/art-20046590

"West Point Grad Battles Eating Disorder"
Retrieved from-
http://abcnews.go.com/Health/Wellness/military-servicemembers-increased-risk-eating-disorders/story?id=15542551
Feb. 8, 2012

Stunkard, AJ. "Eating Disorders and Obesity". *Psychiatr Clin N Am.* 2011; 34(34):765-771.

Whitney, E. N., Cataldo, C. B., & Rolfes, S. R. (1994). *Understanding Normal & Clinical Nutrition.* 4th edition. St. Paul, MN: West Publishing Company.

Jha, P., M.D., Ramasundarahettige, C ., M.Sc., Landsman, V., Ph.D., Rostron, B., Ph.D., Thun, M., M.D., Anderson, R. N., Ph.D., ..., and Peto, R., F.R.S. "1st-Century hazards of smoking and benefits of cessation in the United States." *N Engl J Med* 2013; 368:341-350 January 24, 2013DOI: 10.1056/NEJMsa1211128

Boyle, P. A., Buchman, A. S., Wilson, R. S., Yu, L., Schneider, J. A., and Bennett, D. A. "Effect of Purpose in Life on the Relation Between Alzheimer Disease Pathologic Changes on Cognitive Function in Advanced Age." Arch Gen Psychiatry, May 2012; 69: 499 - 504.

"Exercising Regularly Increases Life Span Even If Overweight"
    Retrieved from-http://www.medicalnews today.com/articles/252464.php

Moore S.C., et al. "Leisure Time Physical Activity of Moderate to Vigorous Intensity and Mortality: A Large Pooled Cohort Analysis." *PLoS Medicine.* November 6, 2012. doi: 10.1371/journal.pmed.1001335.

"Antioxidants: MedlinePlus"
    Retrieved from-http://www.nlm.nih.gov/ medlineplus/antioxidants.html

"Dietary Supplement Fact Sheet: Selenium"
Retrieved from-http://ods.od.nih.gov/
Factsheets/Selenium-Health
Professional

"Lycopene – The World's Healthiest Foods"
Retrieved from-http://www.whfoods.com
/genpage.php?tname=nutrient&dbid=
121

Step 8: Leisure

"Importance of Leisure & Recreation for
Health"
Retrieved from-http://www.livestrong
.com/article/438983-what-are-the-health
-benefits-of-leisure-recreation/

White, E. G. (1942) *The Ministry of Healing*,
Mountain View, CA: Pacific Press.

"14 Things Successful People Do on
Weekends"
Retrieved from-
http://www.forbes.com/sites/jacquelyns
mith/2013/02/22/14-things-successful-
people-do-on-weekends/2/

Clip Art/Photo Images

Following Clip Art/Photo Images retrieved
from- www.publicdomainpictures.net:

Hammock Between Palm Trees. Clip Art by
Karen Arnold; *Pouring Sugar into Tea.* Photo
by Alice Birkin; *Running Man Silhouette.* Clip

Your company or organization may be interested in our trainings:

- ✪ Weigh Less or Pay More
- ✪ Tough Talks- Handling Crucial Conversations Effectively
- ✪ Move From Mediocrity to Achieve Excellence
- ✪ Conflict Resolution
- ✪ ARMY WELL - 8 Steps to Total Wellness
- ✪ Managing Stress Inside Out
- ✪ Manage Me Manage You – Healthy Ways to Lead Others

Call for more information:
Health Opera, LLC.
256-721-4063. visit our website:
www.healthopera.biz

INDEX

www.ingramcontent.com/pod-product-compliance
Lightning Source LLC
Chambersburg PA
CBHW060900280326
41934CB00007B/1122